## Acclaim for *Prickly Cactus*

"This powerful narrative takes the reader through the author's reconnecting and recreating what is most essential to healing and to living: community, tradition, and beliefs, which lead to wholeness of mind, body, and spirit. Professor Delgado Gaitan offers not only a health narrative, but a love story — a journey to self-appreciation, self-care and self-love."

> — Yvette G. Flores, Ph. D., Licensed Clinical Psychologist, Flores Consulting and Psychotherapy

"Candid, courageous testimony about tragedy, challenge, and resilience. It is not only about the body, but about spirit, mind, community, and family. While the author chronicles her many losses, her strong spirit, undaunted hope, and openness to an array of healing possibilities inspire us to seek our own courage and optimism. Prickly Cactus *is a vivid, intimate, and compelling account of Concha Delgado Gaitan's struggle with chronic illness, and the life lessons she learned in the healing process. Bravo!"*

> — Professor Perry Gilmore, University of Arizona, Tucson

Prickly Cactus

Finding Sacred Meaning In Chronic Illness

Concha Delgado Gaitan, Ph.D.

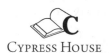

CYPRESS HOUSE

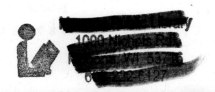

Acknowledgments

With gratitude, I recognize the many loving people who have traveled with me through my healing—my parents, Juan and Maria Delgado; my husband, Dudley Thompson; my sisters' families, the Contreras family; the Vargas family; the Godinez family; and the Estrada family. You edify me.

I have been immensely privileged to have so many friends who have generously extended themselves in so many important ways to create a supportive community. I list them alphabetically except where they are couples: José and Judy Alva, Martha Allexsaht-Snider, Ken and Donna Barnes, Harriet and Craig Buchanan, Nathan Butler, Lubna Chaudhry, Camilo Chavez, Ed DeAvila and Patricia Perez-Arce, Luis and Patty DelAguila and family, Cathy Edgett, Berta Gharrity and family, Perry Gilmore, Nancy Greenman, Berta Gonzalez, Mary Jonlick, Nelva Leivitt and family, Josefina Lopez, Gloria Loventhal and Richard Pederson, Shirley Nakao, Rosemary Papa and Ric Brown, Cindy Pease-Alvarez, Beatriz Pesquera, David Quijada, Marina Rolink, Sandra Schecter, Yolanda Singh, David Smith, Susan Raeburn and Bill Delaney, Sue Tamura, Yolanda Ronquillo, Olga Terrazas, Chalmer Thompson, Toni Vincent, and Karen Watson-Gegeo. And, of course, my book group: Freidel Cohen, Emily Douglas, Beverly Freeman, Meg Hillier, Bonnie Kraus, Irene Kan, Carol Lloyd, Jean Milton, Marta Tanrikulu, Melanie

Tervelon, Renata Tervelon, and Julie Yokoyama. Your friendship animates me.

Countless other friends, too many to list, have kept me smiling by offering good thoughts and prayers on my behalf. For that, I am profoundly appreciative because we know it all works!

Without the superb expertise of my healers from Eastern and Western traditions, this story would not be. They were my rheumatologist, physiatrist, doctor of family practice, urologist, and physical therapists, as well as various doctors of Chinese medicine and the curanderas (Mexican herbal and faith healers). With great respect, I acknowledge your gifts and withhold names to protect your privacy. I will name some of the healers on my team: Luis DelAguila, psychologist—Inner-Path Ministry; Ralph Ortiz, chiropractor; Claramae Weber, nurse and practitioner of Healing Touch Energy Medicine; Amy Lee, acupuncturist, and Karyn Sanders, herbalist and founder of the Blue Otter School of Herbal Medicine. I admire your commitment.

Some have shared their editorial gift of words by reading versions of the manuscript in the making and have helped me to move the project along. Thank you Lisa Zuré, Sandy Little, Sande Smith, Debra Ratner, Nikki Agee, and Marilyn McGuire. Your words empower me.

Although this is an autobiographical narrative, in order to preserve privacy, I omitted, altered, or gave pseudonyms to some people and places in the story.

Introduction

Chihuahua, Mexico's high desert, is home to a vast assortment of cacti. Cacti typically grow slowly, wrapping their roots around rocks to brave the strong winds that blow across their landscape. Chihuahua is also my birthplace. For much of my life I have been surrounded by cacti either as houseplants, medicine, or food. Some cacti are smooth to the touch; others are more prickly. *Nopales* (cacti) provide a substance that is excellent for many medicinal purposes, especially for reducing high blood pressure. The *nopal* is also a vegetable. Cut up, it makes a great accompaniment to scrambled eggs and chorizo—a favorite of mine.

When I became severely ill and disabled with systemic lupus erythematosus (SLE), I pursued strength and balance through memories of my grandma's garden when I was young. Images of summers spent at her house in East Los Angeles flooded me. She tended a thriving *nopal* garden with all the love and care that she gave to everyone she knew. The *nopal* used in Mexican cuisine is externally thorny and untouchable, but its sweet fruit, the prickly pear, reveals its true nature, its mysterious strength—if we're willing to cut through the resilient exterior to the soulful, nutritious interior. And like the prickly cactus, life presents us with thorny challenges, but if we're willing to cut through the prickly exterior, we reach the core lessons that may teach us a great deal about ourselves.

prickly cactus

a body maps its history
in aches and bliss
but we are not our body's sickness
nor muscle strength
nor the reams of paper called work
a body is an altar
where relationships take sanctuary
on crowded layers of success
on imperfections cast as failures
the sun's rays undress its essence
that mimics a stately prickly cactus
thorny at the touch
and wholesome in its roots

Writing in my personal journal, I cut through the thorny parts of my experience and discovered a soothing balm beneath the surface. I compiled this story using personal journals, medical reports, and many readings. I organized it according to salient themes that intersected in my life, shaping the lessons I learned in making meaning of a disabling illness. I describe a life's work crossing borders to learn about new communities, their languages, and cultures.

Some of the lessons that later shaped my healing began early in childhood. I begin the story with childhood, recounting early years, and integrating education with making successful career choices. Later becoming physically unwell, I initiated healing processes that continue in the present.

Living in an immigrant family, I developed a strong identity while learning to value education, work, and faith. I acquired not only a new language but also a new culture. Then, I worked as a teacher, school principal, professor, researcher, and anthropologist in education, which moved me into poor and immigrant families and communities that sometimes resembled the one in which I grew up. As my health declined, I crafted a new language, culture and identity to make sense of this challenge.

Writing this book was a natural extension of the difficult times I faced. I wanted to put a frame around this healing period. During the time when I was quite ill, the researcher in me felt compelled to write daily records and to read extensively about the way an illness affects not only the physical but also the emotional, spiritual, professional, social, and economic changes occurring in my world. Learning to heal meant experimenting with healing modalities and traditions involving mind, body, and spirit. Through it all, I sought meaning in the events that unfolded, more profoundly than ever before. The illness changed me. How I viewed healthy work and relationships changed. Before, I believed I had to recover so that I could again return to work and overextend myself. Now I believe that health is my life's work. The difference is living consciously, finding a balance.

Many people in health crises feel an acute need to transform their situation. My story speaks to both men and women, but more strongly to women. More women are diagnosed with autoimmune diseases, which may share common symptoms. Everyone who suffers chronic and acute pain will appreciate reading of how I recognized the gifts contained within adversity.

Not only is this story of a woman's recovery encouraging, but the multiple conventional and complementary healing traditions are noteworthy both for those who actually have painful chronic diseases and for their supporters and caretakers, who comprise yet another audience.

A broader audience includes men and women who are interested in seeing women transform their lives through overcoming adversity. This story speaks to readers who want to learn how illness can serve as one of life's teachers. Although *Prickly Cactus* is not a formula "how-to" book, it has a very practical message: the healing process consists of three major keys — building supportive community, practicing spirituality, and re-creation.

Believing that telling our story liberates us and heals us, I felt compelled to put pen to paper. The writer Arthur W. Frank says that when people turn their illness into stories, they find healing.[1] And redeeming those prickly parts of our experience happens as we connect with one another through our story.

CHAPTER 1

Reminiscing

Without language to think and talk about our situation,
we cannot give either illness or healing a voice.

There it was, the corner house with that perfectly pruned apple tree. It marked the midpoint on my daily walk. In the fall, crisp Fuji apples overload its branches. One fall day, the owner offered me some when I walked past. Now, in mid-spring the apples are barely blossoms.

Today, as I turned the corner, I heard a cheerful hello. It was the owner. She was moving the water hose on the other side of the tree.

"Finally, we're getting good walking weather," I said.

"You're lucky you can walk," she commented. I thought, If she only knew how much more than luck it has taken to be able to walk. Just then, I felt her presence closer to me along the sidewalk. "I'm Sandy," she introduced herself.

"Nice to meet you," I said. "I'm Concha." Holding and massaging her arms, she began walking gingerly up to her front path, saying to me, "You look so healthy and strong. Enjoy your walk."

As I walked away I fought the urge to tell her that it had taken years for me to be able to walk this far. I hesitated because, after all, I didn't know her. Sandy was just a nice woman who once offered me apples from her tree. My bolder part won. I pivoted back a few steps and called to her as she walked up to her door. "I am grateful that I can walk, but it's taken years for me to do it without wheelchairs, crutches, and canes."

"Do you mind if I ask what kind of illness you have?"

"I was diagnosed with a systemic lupus."

"Oh, my God. I have an autoimmune illness too," Sandy said. "It keeps me in a great deal of pain."

"I understand pain all too well," I replied, "because even now I'm in pain constantly."

Sandy described her situation: "I've been in so much pain that I had to quit working. And without any benefits, I've gone through my savings. There wouldn't be a roof over our heads if not for my mother's generosity."

"I'm very grateful for the angels around me, like family and friends," I said.

"Most of the time, I can't get out of bed. Because of the pain, I haven't been able to find a job that I can do," she said.

"I had to change careers during one of the most critical relapses," I replied. "Typing one letter at a time from bed, I retrained myself to do technical writing from home. I can pace the workday better."

"Oh yes, pace, pace, pace," Sandy echoed, as though she had heard the word quite often.

Pacing, or as my doctor introduced it to me, "alternating activity with rest," was a new concept for me when I became ill. It became part of the healing language I had to learn. Apparently, Sandy, too, had discovered the importance of pacing.

Framing this healing snapshot, I can share with others how to liberate ourselves from a crisis. Despite how our bodies look and feel, we can liberate ouselves from crisis. Essentially, healing occurs as we are able to talk about our illness and healing — and ultimately to connect with the healer within us, with loved ones, including the Sandys around us who support us as we support them.

For years, my muscles and joints ached and burned with pain, commanding unrelenting attention. The pain's ferocious grip persisted until I listened to its lessons. A crying body led me to the young immigrant girl I was, who was filled with excitement about learning English and a new culture, yet who was also traumatized by some of its unfriendly ambassadors. Childhood core values of education and faith were the foundation for social justice work. They built stairs leading me into successful careers, but those stairways fell and crumbled in the face of my health crisis.

CHAPTER 2

Speaking the Mother Tongue

Cuando Dios cierra una puerta abre otras
(When God closes one door he opens others).

Growing up in Mexico holds special memories. When I close my eyes, I can smell the musty old school building and hear the giggles of girlfriends' voices singing *Naranja Dulce* (Sweet Orange). This and other popular circle games and jingles are etched in the souls of young Mexican children even before they start school. In the classroom, the Spanish alphabet letters pinned neatly above the blackboard formed a background behind the young teacher, whose warm smile greeted us every day. By the second grade in the school that I attended in Chihuahua, I was a star student. I delighted and excelled in reading history books in Spanish.

English became a new challenge in Los Angeles when we legally immigrated to reunite with our relatives. I was excited about our new home. Immediately, I dove into the deep end to learn English as quickly as possible. Still, school made me nervous from the beginning. It didn't help that the teacher punished me until I learned to read to her satisfaction. Fearful and anxious, I missed those days in Mexico, where the language and books were familiar and everyone around me understood when I spoke.

In a new culture, I was acutely aware of the communication transmitted through words, actions, and silence. Months passed and conversations with classmates increased. I could say a few things in English: "I like playing with my sisters," and "I like to eat in the cafeteria." But my progress did not impress the teacher, who kept me in during recess for not speaking English well.

Although I could not speak English fluently, I understood quite a bit. One classroom golden rule was "Do not copy your neighbor's paper." This meant that I was not to look at anyone's paper when the teacher instructed us to answer questions in our books. During one incident, I stood up to go to the teacher's desk to ask Mrs. Brown a question. I walked up to tell her that I did not understand the story or the questions in the book. She looked at me and responded, "I've already explained it. You have to answer the questions." I felt humiliated. I returned to my desk and looked around the room, wishing I could see the answers written on my classmates' foreheads. Instead, I saw a sea of blond heads tipped forward reading their books.

Lost for answers, I looked across the aisle to a girl who appeared to know what she was doing. I wanted to shout out to her, "How do you do this? I don't understand what these questions are asking." Just then, I felt the teacher's presence next to me. She stood by my desk. "Let me have your paper," she demanded. I handed it to her, crushed with humiliation as I watched her tear up the clean sheet of paper on which I'd had only enough time to write my name in the upper right-hand corner.

There I sat, alone at my desk, having just learned what it meant to "do your own work." This was individualism, working by oneself, not looking to others for support, and feeling failure if you could not succeed on your own. I had just stepped into the fast lane of the American road to independence.

Most of the time, school traumatized me. I felt nervous just walking onto the grounds. This feeling worsened once I was in the classroom. I wanted so much to show Mrs. Brown that I was trying as hard as I could. When she walked toward me, all I saw was an older woman with salt-and-pepper hair pulled tight in a bun. Her dull eyes showed no compassion. I felt like her captive, scared that she would tell my parents I was not a good student.

Fearing that I would be forever stuck in these feelings, I was determined not to let her get the better of me. I thought, *I know how to read. I'll show you, lady!* Right there and then I promised myself that I would successfully brave this unfriendly place called school. Eventually I did. I learned that schooling had different languages; one of them encouraged learning and the other discouraged it.

Mrs. Brown's intentions might have been sincere, but they did not feel that way to me. Later, I would spend a great deal of time in school, getting a number of academic degrees and researching language and literacy in communities. Mrs. Brown never knew that many years later, when I became a teacher, I would think about her and know that I wanted to teach differently than she had.

Although my mother, Maria, did not speak English very well,

her language was kindness. She'd show up at school on those occasional Fridays with arms full of chocolate cupcakes for our class. She became a room mother and helped the teachers at every class gathering. Everyone loved Mom. Her visits to the classroom were important to me; I felt I belonged.

My mother set high expectations for my four sisters and me. She modeled discipline, strength, hard work, and faith in her strict but nurturing way. Her loving style of parenting balanced my father's authoritarian role in the family. Her words about the importance of *"educación"* made a strong impression on me. *Educación* has a much broader meaning for me than its English translation, "education." *Educación* encompasses how we comport ourselves in life. To be *"una persona educada"* (an educated person) means getting a formal education, being respectful, and having good manners. It implies a willingness to cooperate and to peacefully coexist with others. I worked hard to avoid being caught behaving selfishly because Mom would say, *"Asi no se comporta una persona con educación."* (An educated person doesn't behave that way.)

My mother's faith in my ability made it possible to believe in myself. Her belief that respecting others was part of being an educated person shielded me from the sting of discrimination when classmates ridiculed me because I was Mexican or because I did not speak English very well. Knowing the difference between *educación* and education, I dismissed unfriendly comments. I stayed open to friendships that nurtured me.

Mom worked at home, taking care of us. Our house in Los Angeles was one large room that served as a kitchen (with a small sink, a tiny stove, a mini-refrigerator), as two bedrooms (divided by a curtain), and a rest area with a couch. We had a black-and-white TV that we watched only an hour a night.

The bathroom was small but it did have a door. Mom kept our house as comfortable as possible.

Surrounding the house was a small yard next to the driveway where my sisters and I played. Calla lilies, geraniums, and thick white daisy bushes encircled a patch of neatly mowed green lawn in front. In these surroundings, I had many opportunities to practice English. Although I preferred to speak English so that I could talk with friends, Spanish was the family language at home.

Issues of the body and health were frequent topics of conversation in the family because in our vast extended family, someone was always sick. An aunt died of cancer. Mom had frequent bouts of pneumonia. A younger sister often had migraine headaches. Mom and Dad believed that sickness and problems of the body were inevitable.

All the talk about illness scared me, but when I actually fell or got a scrape, Mom made it all better. Mexican parents have a rhyme that they tell their young ones when they are hurt or do not feel well. It goes, "*Sana, sana, colita de rana, si no se sana hoy se sanara mañana.*" It's a cheerful verse affirming that you will heal; if it does not heal today, it will heal tomorrow. Typically, an adult says this while holding and stroking the painful part of the child's body.

On Faith

Thinking back, it was probably a black widow that bit me. For sure, it was a mean spider. I screamed, and my sisters, who were playing hide-and-seek with me, came running. Instantly, my foot was swollen and bright red. Mom ran out of the house and rushed to me. She called our neighbor to take us to the hospital emergency room. No time for the traditional mustard patches that Mom religiously used with a cup of homegrown *yerbabuena* (mint) tea that allayed every physical ailment. I was scared, even though the doctor was very nice as he popped the large, pus-filled blister. The doctor kept me in the hospital for a couple of days until the fever broke. Mom and Dad visited every evening. Mom gave me a small medallion of the Virgin Mary, saying that it would protect me.

I knew about saints and prayer. One lasting memory I have is dusting the furniture on Saturdays, being very careful not to disturb Grandmother's altar to the *Virgen de Guadalupe*, her statue surrounded by candles on one corner of the dresser. On its opposite end was Grandfather's statue of Buddha, with one candle in front of it. Grandmother's belief was an indigenous form of Catholicism, typically practiced by many Mexicans; grandpa's came from his Chinese ancestral home.

Long after my grandparents died there were always lit candles around our house—offered up for special occasions to some holy figure.

Prayer was an easy language to master. Every morning I watched Mom stand in front of her altar, which was adorned with her patron saint and candles. She whispered a prayer, then crossed and blessed herself. Then she lit a candle. From the other room, I watched Mom's faith ritual. I remember the feeling of total stillness at that moment as she lit the candle. There is no feeling I can compare to this holy moment when Mom prayed at her altar. At the strike of a match, her lit candle transformed a small room into a sacred space.

At about age nine, clutching the medallion in my hand in that dark hospital room, I prayed the Our Father. Then I fell asleep.

I fell in love with language in his class. New friends and a new setting energized me. I not only joined Finance Club, Spanish Club, the yearbook staff, Thespians, Choir, and Scholarship Society, I also made good friends, achieved scholastically, worked after school, and volunteered in the community.

School is a mix of penalties and rewards, and I experienced both throughout all the grades, but the accolades were the best in my senior year in high school. Mrs. Nichols, the counselor, called me into her office. "You are on the list as one of the top ten of your graduating class." It sounded good to me, not that I'd been competing against anyone; I was simply crazed with learning. I won a gold seal and a $50 cash prize from the PTA. And the winning streak had just begun!

I applied for a $500 scholarship from the scholarship society, but a good friend of mine won it instead. When she received her award, she told me she felt bad for me. She asked, "Are you okay?"

"I'm fine," I said. "I know that God never closes one door without opening another." Mom's words made the most sense to me at the time, and they worked; her wisdom got me through this disappointment, too.

Two weeks later, I received a letter from the University of the Pacific (UOP), where I had applied for admission to their Inter-American Studies Program. UOP offered me a four-year scholarship, which covered tuition and fees. This was a great deal, even though I would have to work for room and board. Work was no stranger to me.

In both Spanish and English, belief in self and strong effort rewarded me. More important than which language I spoke growing up were the messages I heard: to have faith, love my family, achieve academically, remain independent, and never forget to work hard.

a local health clinic that served poor families in our community asked me to become an interpreter after school. The building was the size of a small three-bedroom home. It was clean and whitewashed, with dangling pots of geraniums by the front doors. The doctors were white and spoke only English. Mothers brought their children there even if the appointment was for the mom. Doctors called me in to the examining room when they had a person who had not brought along an interpreter.

Language about medical needs requires some instruction, which I didn't receive. Most of the time, I conveyed the right message to both sides. But translating wasn't as difficult for me as the messages I heard from the doctors about the families they treated. One Wednesday afternoon, only one doctor showed up, and I had to sit in the examining room with him and the nurse while he talked with patients. He smirked every time a patient left the room. I imagined it was a bad habit. Then, when one woman came in with her son, he finished examining them and the nurse left the room. As the woman put on her son's jacket, she looked at me and smiled. She gave the doctor a cursory smile and said, "Thank you." He turned to look at me and then he turned to them, asking me, "Tell them they should cut down on those tortillas. Too fat. They should know better. That's what's making them sick." And he laughed. The woman looked at me, her eyes waiting for an interpretation. I was too shocked to say anything to anyone. I remained quiet and smiled at her, indicating that the doctor's comments were unworthy of translation. "*Que les vaya bien*," I said to her. ("May all go well for you.") But she insisted on knowing what he'd said. "*¿Qué dice de las tortillas?*" ("What's he saying about tortillas?")

I replied, "*Dice que cuando come uno muchas que causan gordura.*" ("He says that when one eats too many tortillas, they cause overweight.") The doctor turned to write in the file.

"*Digalé que yo no les doy mucho que comer.*" ("Tell him that I don't overfeed my family.") She walked out the door.

I told the doctor what she had said. He just smirked.

He could have been talking about our family. Some of us were a bit overweight, but it wasn't because Mom overfed us. She was quite conscious about what we ate. Despite that, some of us have battled weight issues throughout our lives.

This doctor had missed his opportunity to do his job. Where he needed to connect, he rejected. Where he needed to teach, he ridiculed. I felt I needed to help protect the patients from this doctor. I lacked the words to tell him that he needed to change and help the families with education, with resources, and with understanding.

Fortunately, many of these unspoken injustices found a voice on the street through the chants of protesters and the banners they carried, demanding an end to poverty conditions as well as an end to the Vietnam War. As often as possible, I joined my generation in marches and protests calling attention to every cause demanding social change in our society. Dialogues exploded in the street, producing an exchange of diverse ideas, challenging us to understand different points of view. We were the baby boomers — born after WW II — now exercising our political strength with cries for a just and peaceful world. Inspired and challenged by the words and works of President John F. Kennedy, Martin Luther King, Cesar Chavez, and Mohandas Gandhi to create a moral and nonviolent world, we had the political climate on our side.

On Saturday morning, August 29, 1970, my sister Carmen and

I were at our parents' home, back from college. We planned to join our friends in a park in East Los Angeles to march down Whittier Blvd. in the National Chicano Moratorium March against the Vietnam War. Fast-forward to more current times and the newspaper headlines might read LATINOS MARCH TO PROTEST WAR IN IRAQ.

That first large Chicano protest of its kind happened on one of the hottest, smoggiest summer days in Los Angeles. My sister Carmen and I got up at dawn, wanting to leave the house as early as possible. "Do you know exactly where we're meeting the Chicano group from Cal State?" I asked her, grabbing one of Mom's soft, warm, perfectly round flour tortillas from the basket on the kitchen table as we headed out the back screen door.

"On the south side of Belvedere Park," Carmen said.

I tossed her the keys. "You know where we're going, so you drive."

"Let's just get out of here before Mom and Dad figure out where we're going. You know how they hate for us to go to marches," Carmen said.

"Do you have your gas mask?"

"What are you talking about?"

"Have you seen how those cops throw tear gas at the antiwar marchers? They're not going to like thousands of Chicanos in East Los Angeles demonstrating against the war."

"What's so radical about ending the war and spending the money on poor people who need it?"

"Nothing. Let's just go," I urged.

Blocks away, we could hear drumbeats pounding and chants blaring from every corner of the park. People who waved signs with different slogans were united in only one message: "Stop the war in Vietnam!"

Along with 30 thousand other demonstrators, we marched the six-mile stretch between Belvedere Park and Laguna Park in East LA. *Virgen de Guadalupe* banners waved freely throughout the sea of marchers. In the US, the *Virgen de Guadalupe* was an icon that represented the spirit of liberation. The *Virgen* carried a timeless message: we are all one. She was a strong presence in our home; she was not only Mexico's patron saint, but also Grandma's and Dad's. In spite of my familiarity with this icon, I didn't relate to spiritual figures during this period. In a paradoxical way, I rejected the religious aspect of Mexican culture while wanting to change the oppressive conditions in poor communities. Although I respected liberation theology and believed that the liberal wing of the Catholic Church should lead the movement to correct injustice in poor communities, work had by then become the obsession in my life that I most trusted.

From local to national political arenas, my activism taught me that poverty was born of unequal economic conditions, not of people's personal choice. Just as poverty is created, it can be eased when people have access to education and a political voice. Our national leaders, including Doctor King and Cesar Chavez, championed these ideals through spiritual currents. Although their political discourse inspired me, other political voices discouraged belief in religious practices among activists; religion was considered "the opiate of the people." As I looked around the world, the countries where religion dominated were where the poorest people were found. My belief that religion oppressed the poor actually discounted the social and economic origins of poverty. That religion sustained people day by day did not concern me then. Only later did I come to understand that religion itself did not create poverty. I now

believe my early view was an arrogant and disrespectful attitude that dismissed people's spiritual beliefs as misguided
and wrong.

Despite my disregard for others' beliefs, I continued march-
ing side by side with those holding *Virgen de Guadalupe* banners, as I respected their choosing to wave their faith. Block
after block we marched. Finally, we could see Laguna Park
ahead. With a parched throat I chanted along with everyone,
"US out of Vietnam!" and "What do we want? Peace! When do
we want it? Now!" Suddenly word spread through the march
that there was trouble ahead at the park. We heard that Ruben
Salazar, a journalist for the Los Angeles Times and KMEX-TV,
had been killed by the police.

Five hundred policemen swept the park, swinging clubs
and hurling tear-gas grenades. Panic erupted. Some people
began breaking the windows of businesses along Whittier
Boulevard.

"Quick, run up this street!" Carmen screamed to me, grabbing my forearm. I looked back to see if our friends followed.
They ran behind us down the side street. We kept running away
from Whittier until we all caught a bus heading in the opposite direction from the turmoil.

Three others besides Ruben Salazar were killed and three
hundred were injured that day. The investigation into Salazar's
death absolved the Los Angeles police of any wrongdoing, fur-
ther widening the divide between Chicanos and the police, but
strengthening the Chicano community's voice for justice. The
frightening events of Saturday, August 29, fueled our resolve to
change unjust conditions and continue protesting the war.

Los Angeles was only one spot in a nationwide frenzy to
change the political and cultural landscape. All across the

country, change percolated in every level of society. This forced gender roles to change in the workplace and in our homes. Many of us found our personal lives turned inside out by the demands of our activism while working full-time on our careers and completing university degrees.

It seemed as if questioning my role as a woman in this society had been going on from the beginning. I had a mom who tried to inculcate solid Mexican values in us while also encouraging us to learn to succeed in our new culture. And Mom achieved her goal—she raised five strong, intelligent, and professionally successful women.

Mom wrestled with her own desire for independence and the roles she played as a wife and mother. Yet her counsel made a lasting impact upon her daughters: "Getting married is a choice. Having children is a choice. Taking your husband's name is a choice. But you had better have your own checkbook, because that's the only way you'll have freedom." I concluded that Mom was a feminist long before it was popular to claim that identity. For me, there seemed to be no contradiction in having it all; I wanted a successful career and a loving relationship while continuing to work as a community activist.

The reality of straddling career, personal relationship, and political activism was a daunting challenge. At home, my relationship with my partner, Robert, had been stressful from the start. I struggled to balance the demands of working on a master's degree and full-time teaching, while dealing with his difficult disposition. Finally, Robert's lack of support for me became exhausting. His demanding temperament collided with my ardent resistance to acquiesce to traditional gender roles. We found ourselves two migrants under the same roof. Unable to reconcile our differences, and tired of Stockton's dense fog, I

gift for all occasions where a present was expected. The book taught us that caring for our bodies was part of our liberation and responsibility. Decisions involving our bodies, including pregnancy, abortion, and childcare became major political public-health issues as well as political platforms. *Our Bodies, Ourselves* did not, however, address the daily care of our bodies, including the relationship between overwork, stress, and chronic illness. In fairness to the publication, the current edition of the book contains updates on chronic illnesses prevalent among women.

Working intensely, I became accustomed to focusing on external responsibilities while ignoring their impact on my body and health. This was possible through self-discipline, instilled by parental modeling and professional training. When I was preparing to become a teacher, I was accepted in the first undergraduate Teacher Corps. Its mission was to make us teacher-trainees change agents in the school. The message was not something I could limit to the schools where I worked. I usually met my students and their families in their homes weeks before school began in September. I wanted to make sure that the parents understood the classroom program and what I expected of them.

Whether in the classroom or in the streets, change came through right thinking, right action, and physical endurance that kept us in meeting after meeting, boycott after boycott, and protest march after march. The only work I had patience for was that which showed tangible changes in people's lives. Did families have a roof over their heads? Did the children I taught have shoes without holes? Did adults in the community have employment? Work was the top priority. I had to count on my body more than ever before to do a good job in the school as well as in the political work. I felt responsible for making change happen; all I could count on was my physical strength and my intelligence. At that time, I expected that physical stamina would sustain me. There was no room for belief or spiritual practice. Problems had only concrete solutions, according to political orientations that trusted only the material world. In later years, I recognized the error of my ways: I could not expect to change external conditions without also changing my inner spirit.

In my mid-twenties, creating social change was the main goal in educational and political work. I walked out of the classroom and into the principal's office — the first woman principal ever hired in that district. As I walked into my new school, I was filled with demanding messages daily: "Do more. Do it better. Do it faster." I had set the bar at an impossible height. I not only had a demanding principalship in the district's largest elementary school, which was also an academically high-risk school, but also took leadership positions in statewide committees for the development of curriculum frameworks. All of it seemed worthwhile as long as I could walk around the playground and talk with the children; they took my hand and said, "I want to grow up and be a principal, too."

Innovation and change shaped our vision in that school; continuously, I organized workshops for the staff and for parents to learn how to improve children's learning.

"Those of us going to the Herb Kohl Learning Center in Point Arena need to be here on Friday afternoon at 3:30 p.m. sharp," I instructed the staff.

"What's on the agenda when we get there?" one teacher asked.

"We'll cook dinner with Herb's family and he'll give us an

orientation for the literacy workshop that'll follow for Saturday and Sunday." I explained.

"Will we have a chance to take a walk on the beach or around his ranch?" another teacher asked.

"You will, but those of us planning the agenda will have to put in quite a bit of time," I clarified.

As an educational leader, my strongest concern was to maximize our knowledge and skills to best serve children and their families. Change in the school came at a great expense. My days of bike riding, playing tennis and dancing were fewer. Everything and everyone at the school received my time and attention, leaving me exhausted and occasionally feeling depleted emotionally.

Working Through Dark Places

Sometimes work protects us from feeling pain in our bodies and our lives. We look for shelters and befriend denial until we're handed a situation impossible to ignore. As stressful as work was, I sometimes preferred dealing with the demands of the office to grappling with personal relationships. Paul, my life-partner, and I had been on and off for some time. Our issues could probably be traced to our patterns of overwork as we tried to build our careers. At some point, the pressure at the office became intolerable. Then I began listening to my gut sense that adamantly called for a career change.

I left administration to pursue a doctorate at Stanford University. Before starting the doctoral program, however, I took a slight detour—becoming a mommy. My hopes were that motherhood would inspire a gentler pace in my life, time for my loved ones, and maybe an occasional day off, priorities

I had omitted in the shuffle of work. However, my new-laid plans were not to be.

My mind still goes crazy when I remember the birth of my daughter Maya. I wish I could wave a wand and undo what happened at San Francisco General Hospital. It is a giant old building, but the alternative birth center was cozy and comfortable. Maya was a beautiful, fair-skinned little six-pound baby with thick, straight, black hair. I looked at her and recalled thinking how my nieces and nephews were born with lots of hair all over, not just the head. I held Maya close, but they took her from me quickly. Something went terribly wrong.

What followed is like a dense fog now. My obstetrician came into the room. Paul held me. "They don't know exactly what went wrong," the doctor said. "She bled internally. It's rare, but we've seen it before. It happens once in every 20,000 births with twins. But yours was a single birth. It's a mystery. Maya died."

I heard it, but I thought maybe they had drugged me and I was hallucinating.

"That's not possible!" I screamed. I lay sobbing.

Death was a big part of our lives, as is the case when you're part of a large family: I had lost grandparents, aunts, uncles, cousins, and friends, but nothing I knew before had prepared me for this. It was foreign territory, where even questions failed me. I felt dead in mind, body, and spirit.

There it was—a shattered piece of my life. And I felt like a failure because I couldn't fix it. I had no option left but to turn inward, to hide from everything that had once seemed important. For someone who once believed that education could solve everything, I was now facing a major reality: no amount of schooling, even a doctorate degree, could change what happened. I lost all sense of self. The funny part was that I didn't know what that self was that I had lost. I just knew that I felt empty, my identity unknown. How would I make it one day to the next? What awaited would involve discovering what lay beneath the numb part of me.

Couples who are unable to deal with the grief and stress of losing a child often separate. Following Maya's death, Paul and I became a statistic along with over 90% of parents in this situation. Now it's just me, I thought, alone with the lump in my throat. The stillness in the house tormented me to tears daily. The only word that my mind understood was "work." I dove headfirst into my doctoral studies. They made sense. I could count the number of pages I read and the papers I wrote. They were tangible.

Doctoral work at Stanford was the perfect medicine. It masked every feeling I once had. But it was only an escape while I worked in the library or studied with others in study groups. For an entire year after Maya's death, there was no hiding from myself when I was alone. In recurring nightmares, I saw myself talking to one of my sisters or a childhood friend who had given birth to twins. The woman with twins gave me one of her babies. I was thrilled. Suddenly, the dream changed. A man pursued me with a knife or gun. I fled for my life in a desperate chase. I hid in a cave or an empty building for protection. The chase ended when the pursuer startled me and threatened my life. I woke up screaming, drenched in perspiration.

I felt like I had fallen off the tightrope and someone had forgotten to put out the net. "I need to believe in something," I said to my friend Irene.

"You believe in many things. You've had such successful careers. That's why you're always so busy."

"I want something I can trust to make me feel safe."

"Are you dreaming? No one has that."

"I did, when I was a kid."

"That was you being a child."

I yearned for faith and rituals from simpler days to fill the emptiness. Having abandoned Catholicism years before, I continued to turn to academic work for comfort, but it never came. In solitude at home, I momentarily pushed aside my books and dissolved into tears. Then I began judging the tears. I thought, I should not feel this way. That's enough crying. I have to work. If I were truly strong, I wouldn't let this loss hurt me. If I let myself hurt, I'll be abandoning my strong self.

But I had it all wrong. If I'd let myself hurt, I wouldn't have turned against myself. Turning against myself was easy in the isolation I created. As long as I didn't allow myself to feel the hurt, I wasn't allowing myself to be a complete person. A whole person experiences the good and the painful.

Most people who got a hint of what was happening to me said, "Get busier." Only a couple of friends knew my pain. Sonia broke the chain. She insisted that I find a community that supported my spiritual healing. She said, "You need to go see a practitioner at the Church of Religious Science."

"No church for me!" I responded adamantly.

"Religious Science is a church where they hold meditation sessions and grief-support groups," she responded.

In reality, I was afraid that I was burdening Sonia with my emotional needs. She piqued my curiosity enough to attend. That Wednesday evening I sat in the small fellowship hall, several rows from the front. I didn't want to appear too interested. I wanted to be invisible this first time. A group of ten had gathered. From the beginning, the music and reassuring words transported me to a land beyond time. I felt a joy that had been dormant for what seemed like an eternity. It was like opening a window that had been painted shut and finding the "something" that would make me feel safe.

Once again I looked forward to another day, feeling that I could trust something bigger than the wounded part of me. This was a new language, and my journal became my partner. Curled up in bed before turning off the light, I scribbled down the events of the day. Confronted by the truth of what I felt, I could release the harsh judgments I'd held against myself.

Our historical and cultural times play strongly in the events in our lives. The '80s exploded with movements pointing us inward, reminding us that we are more than our bodies. The inner child, spirituality, and the afterlife made their popular debut in books and seminars. They invited us to explore the inner spirit. Thank goodness for the timing. On some level, I felt comforted that there were resources for dealing with my pain. Most local bookstores devoted at least one shelf to the topic of death and grief. I was a frequent patron at all of them. It wasn't difficult to find the major authors.

Learning the language for healing my pain of loss was different from any job I'd ever held, any relationship I'd ever had, and any challenge I had ever confronted. I drew on what was available through community, writings, and my own willingness to let my heart see differently.

One afternoon I sat on the tile floor of my favorite bookstore, avidly reading Stephen Levine's book on loss, *Unattended Sorrow: Recovering from Loss and Reviving the Heart*. I couldn't afford to purchase it on a student budget, but I managed to scrape up the money for a ticket to hear his lecture when he came to town. Levine said that loss is painful because we form attachments to people in our lives. In his lecture, Levine shared ideas from his book, arguing that we need to let go of our attachment to each other while we're in this world.[2] Those words hurt as deeply as my loss. What a cynical notion, I thought. I'd rather have my attachment anytime, than let go of my loved ones and pretend that they're dead while they're alive. Walking out of the lecture was my way of rejecting his message.

Heartbreak. How does one ever feel complete again? Mom didn't always have a quick recipe for emotional distress, but she usually had the wisdom to know what I needed. One evening, I sat in the middle of the living room rug, piles of research papers around me; the puddle of tears smeared the print. The phone rang.

"Hello dear," Mom began.

"Hi, Mom. How are you?"

"You sound like you have a cold."

"No. I've had a tough day."

"Dear, I know you have a lot of pressure with your work, but it won't get easier until you make peace with yourself and learn to forgive."

Through sobs, I said, "I know." But I don't really know how, I admitted to myself. What does forgiveness mean anyway? "Whom do I forgive, Mom? Me? Maya? The situation? God?"

"It's you, dear," she said. "You need to know that this is not your fault. Your baby is peaceful now. You need to be peaceful, too."

Forgiveness—each time I did it, it got easier. I found myself needing to do it around every corner. The notion of forgiveness that opened my eyes was that when I forgive myself, the situation had no power over me anymore. No, forgiveness doesn't induce amnesia. After all, we have memory. However, in forgiveness, we take ourselves off the emotional hook, restoring our inner peace.

Even after forgiveness, I continued to peel back the layers of pain. Weekly meditation classes, grief-support groups, lectures, and readings by Virginia M. Satir, Elizabeth Kubler-Ross, and Stephen Levine, as well as Buddhist writings, held me captive when I wasn't busy writing research papers for my classes. Spiritual readings motivated me to join a study group, which met on Fridays. Wearing a black jogging suit, hair pulled back tight, and no make-up, I drove to the community center where I met with a roomful of others dressed in comfortable clothes. We sat on mats on the floor, reading from Buddhist traditions, including *The Miracle of Mindfulness* by Thich Nhat Hanh. A short meditation followed our reading session. Fit and limber, I got into the lotus position; for a short while, time stood still. Inhale. Exhale. One breath at a time. That was all that mattered in the moment. After study group meetings, I felt calm. I understood the course readings without the anxiety that accompanied me.

The more I meditated, the better I could focus on work; drawing boundaries between obsessive work and me became easier. Playing tennis as often as I could on weekends during the day and dancing at nights with friends kept me strong. I could balance work and play. If I didn't stay conscious of my purpose for doing doctoral research, I got sidetracked into the workaholic pace. Fortunately, I had the freedom to study the communities that interested me, making it possible to understand change and social justice among disenfranchised people. Brazilian philosopher and educator Paulo Freire's vision and writings on liberation of poor communities in various parts of the world inspired me.

I first met Freire through his book *Pedagogy for the Oppressed*. The passion behind his thoughts and theories were visible in every word he spoke. At the time that this visionary visited the Bay Area, he was exiled from Brazil for organizing, teaching, and liberating the indigenous poor communities. Then he began traveling the world to carry his message of empowering the oppressed through literacy. A UC Berkeley professor hosted Freire at his home. In a huge two-story Berkeley brown shingle located several blocks from campus, over fifty people crammed into the professor's living room. The Portuguese-speaking man with fair complexion and slightly graying hair sat in a maroon antique chair that seemed to swallow him. The professor facilitated the questions directed to Freire, who answered thoughtfully, pausing frequently in search of the exact English word. We all hung on every word he spoke. One man at the rear of the room called out his question: "How can we use your notions of change to help those who are poor, illiterate, and oppressed here? They are hurting and need homes, jobs, education, and freedom from this oppressive system."

"You begin where they are. What is it that they know? Everyone knows something." We all listened intently. However, before anyone could comment, Freire continued, "You sound very angry. Before you can help others, you must put aside your own anger. Anger is very destructive when you are trying to help others to build their lives."

A pregnant pause followed. His words rang loudly in me, personally and academically. Little else has made such an impact in the way I think about my political work in communities. His wisdom could not have been more timely.

I had heard this before when working for the United Farm Workers. Union leaders espoused Cesar Chavez's philosophy that we should be impatient with the problem but not with our-selves. Maybe I was more mature now and could hear the wis-dom in words that had failed to reach me as profoundly before. I interpreted Freire's words to mean that to empower others, we need to operate from a position of hope, not despair.

That everyone is a whole person regardless of his or her impoverished condition is one of Freire's perspectives that inspired my work. He put into words what I felt deeply when I began investigating and writing about community oral and written traditions. The more I employed Freire's concepts, the more I was able to heal myself through my profession. For the first time, I felt a strong connection between my work and my personal values. Unbeknownst to me, the next time I was to see Freire I would be a professor at UC Santa Barbara, where I sat on a panel with him to discuss family and community lit-eracy research based on his notions of empowerment.

While still at Stanford, I became immersed in research in a northern California community, working with families and children. As I observed the children's play, they taught me their songs and rhymes while all held hands in circle games. Observing and participating in their family rituals and com-munity lore, I learned how their connection through stories kept the children's friendships together.

Working in this community returned me to familiar issues of struggle and liberation. I observed how kids were self-suf-ficient and intelligent at home, but not so in the classroom, where they struggled to follow the rules in a language they barely understood. These children taught me to stay focused on the real reason that I was at Stanford. Research was not a clinical exercise in a laboratory; it was about real people's lives. Through these children and their families, I revisited my past and reclaimed a sense of confidence, determination, and the broader meanings of *educación*.

Four years passed on the road to "moving on" with life and making peace with myself after losing Maya. I finished my doctorate at Stanford and accepted a professorship to teach Anthropology in Education at UC Santa Barbara. I even had a new life partner, Eric. When I took the professorship at UC Santa Barbara, we had to have a commuter relationship. Yes, things had changed, yet part of me felt like I was missing something.

One day I took flowers to Maya's grave, not a frequent trip for me, but on her birthday, August 29, before leaving to assume my new position, I felt inclined to visit. I sat on the damp ground. Quiet. Alone. So I thought. Looking around the forest-green hill, I felt a strong presence approaching my left shoulder. I turned to find an ivory-colored, cloud-shaped, misty form hovering over me. A soft female voice floated in my direction, filling my entire body, telling me, "You are free now. Forgive yourself and go forward." I choked with sobs exploding out of me. I cannot account for the blur in time that followed.

The significance of Maya's birth date was not lost in the spiritual experience of the day: August 29 was also the anniversary of the march in Los Angeles where I had marched to liberate poor communities from oppressive conditions such as illiteracy, poverty, and war. Now, several years later, on August 29, Maya died and liberated herself. In the process, she helped me to forgive and to liberate myself. Her loss reminded me what I had abandoned. I reconnected with that wise, trusting part of me that the young Conchita already knew — the part that held wisdom and knowledge beyond the books I read.

CHAPTER 4

Grappling for Words

*We need to speak about illness, about potential for healing,
and about building supportive communities
around us to transform our lives.*

One advantage of being a professor in the field of Anthropology and Education is that I collaborated with colleagues in parts of the world that I might otherwise never have visited. Alaska was such a place. Working with Alaskan Native students and their communities thrust me into a reality of US history that I had only read about in American Indian writings. Inupiaq elders tell of how their villages were alive with the laughter of children, and then one day, "The planes came. They took the children to Western schools. Many of us still recall the humiliation of standing in the corner of the room and the sting of the ruler across our hands for speaking even one word of Inupiat, our native language."

Years later, the children returned to their villages without their native language and culture. More than time had been lost. Parents and children could not communicate with each other in their native tongue. Without a common language, parents could not teach their culture to their young. The gap had never been wider between generations. Fishing, hunting, and other skills and customs became difficult for villagers to continue.

My friends David Smith and Perry Gilmore were anthropology professors at the University of Alaska, Fairbanks. They invited me to work with Alaskan Native students in a summer research institute. The students had read my books and wanted to employ the research strategies in their respective villages. Shageluk, an Athabaskan village, invited me to work with the teaching staff that was developing a multicultural curriculum in their school. The intent was to teach the students their native language in what they called language regeneration. Once lost, their mother tongue was now being restored through the efforts of the elders and linguists who had taught themselves their native languages.

Flying to Shageluk, I looked out the window of a single-engine mail-drop plane. For two hours, between Anchorage and Shageluk, I looked down on fjords and saw snow-capped mountains that stopped my breath. The plane landed on a strip where three of us deplaned and walked into the village of 200 people.

Alaskans are known for their selfless hospitality. But this I did not expect. As I headed for the schoolhouse, people greeted me by my first name as I passed them on the street. These people, whose history had been silenced for so many years, extended a wonderfully warm welcome to this stranger. I instantly connected with them. In different ways, our respective cultures had experienced learning new languages. The Athabaskans spoke a language of friendship and generosity. Then there was the famous honey-bucket that brought my hosts and me closer together at nights. When I was a young girl, growing up in Mexico without running water, we used a *basinilla* (chamber pot) unless we wanted to go to the outhouse. In Shageluk, without running water, I felt at home.

An added benefit of a place without running water is that it slows down the day's hectic pace. People made eye contact and walked and talked at a gentler pace than ours in large cities. The discussion groups with Alaskan students enriched me. Except for constantly dodging mosquitoes that terrorized me because I developed an allergic reaction to their bite, Alaska anchored me. Its unhurried pace summoned me back for several summers during my professorships at UC Santa Barbara and UC Davis.

After spending five years in Santa Barbara, I was offered a professorship at UC Davis. I couldn't have been happier to live in the Bay Area again. It had always been home for me. Finally Eric and I could reunite. I felt calm. With Eric frequently out of town on business, it was easy for me to recreate the Alaskan tempo. On Sunday mornings, I made a ritual of going to a favorite local café to read the paper with friends. There has never been any shortage of great coffee in the Bay Area. For that, I looked forward to weekends.

One particular weekend I broke my tradition. Feeling exhausted on this early spring Saturday night, I uncharacteristically retired early. At 4:00 a.m. I awoke with shallow breathing. My heart was flipping somersaults and my head was hot to the touch. From shoulders to toes, every muscle and joint screamed with what felt like third-degree-burns coming from inside, searing. Immobilized, I remained in bed. Was this a nightmare? The symptoms intensified. With great effort, I summoned every ounce of strength and crawled to the bathroom.

With no thermometer at hand, I took a Tylenol and splashed water on my body. I was scared as my cheeks got bright red. I was home alone and didn't dare phone to wake anyone. If this were a minor thing, I'd feel foolish if I got anyone out of bed at this hour. After all, taking care of myself was my forte. But could I get myself to the car and drive to the emergency room this time? As I drove to the hospital, my work schedule concerned me the most: if these symptoms persisted, work would be disrupted.

The attending physician looked down my throat and, given all the symptoms, concluded, "You have high fever and body ache. Go home and drink lots of liquid."

I managed to drive home, wondering how I'd even be able to get out of bed to drink fluids. This Sunday morning I would have to skip the Sunday ritual of sipping espresso and reading the Times with friends.

After two days of relentless symptoms, I called my family doctor. He told me to come into the office. Suspecting that I had more than the flu, he ordered lab work. I worried about getting to class that afternoon. After leaving the doctor's office I drove to my office. A typical one-hour commute seemed longer and longer. Halfway to campus, I knew I'd be late for class since I couldn't exert enough pressure to accelerate over 50 mph. By the time I arrived, I was dizzy, exhausted, and felt like I wouldn't be able to get out of the car. In slow motion, I managed to take tiny steps up to the classroom. The class had gone, since students only have to wait twenty minutes for their professor.

The next day, the doctor called and asked me to make another appointment. He announced that the lab results suggested a possible rheumatoid inflammation and referred me to a rheumatologist/immunologist for complete testing.

A week later, when I consulted with Dr. Barrett, the rheumatologist, I had lost ten pounds and was already walking with a cane. Dr. Barrett, a woman of medium height, dressed elegantly and had a strong professional demeanor. Though she spoke sternly, she had a caring heart, which I noticed increasingly with each visit. She listened attentively and with compassion to my story, writing copious notes about my medical history as I detailed my body's daily drama. She ordered the ANA test, a skin biopsy, and myriad other tests.

For two weeks while I waited for the results, I pretended to conduct my normal day-to-day routine as a professor. My body was present, but my mind was absent—busy worrying about what was happening to my body. The day that I returned to Dr. Barrett for the biopsy results, I could think of nothing else. In her office, she pulled up a chair and sat next to me. Holding the lab reports in hand, she explained the statistical patterns. It sounded like a foreign language. I wanted to scream, "Tell me what all this means and let me out of here!" But she continued, carefully showing me the statistical distribution in the various lab tests. Finally, she concluded, "The statistics aren't glaring, but given the speckled pattern that is present, the positive skin biopsy, your hair loss, fatigue, and pained joints, not to mention your medical history of rheumatic fever, I have no choice but to treat your case as systemic lupus erythematosus."

I sat erect. Stoic. It's called denial. Then I felt a glimmer of hope, thinking that surely there must be strong drugs available to solve the problem.

"What's going to happen?" I asked.

"Lupus is a tissue disease that can affect many different

systems. Sometimes symptoms are less acute and at other times more severe."

It didn't matter what they called this thing that was happening to my body. "I'm going to prescribe steroids and hope they reduce the inflammation and pain," she said. "If not, then I'll have to put you on Lukeran, an oral chemotherapy drug used for some patients with autoimmune illnesses."

None of what she said made any sense to me, nor did it matter much. The burning question was, "Will I ever be able to feel well again and walk without a cane?" I missed half of the doctor's explanation as I wandered to how this could affect my life.

I went directly to the library to research medical books. The repeated refrain in everything I read was that there was no cure for this disease but the symptoms could be treated with drugs. Lots of medical terminology and statistics made the deluge of information feel like an academic exercise. I promised myself that I would not be a victim to the symptoms that the publications described. After all, my name was Concha, which means shell. A shell can be delicate, like a seashell, or tough like that of a turtle's back. And I knew which concha I was — strong, iron-like. There I sat, fatigued, with my muscles and joints burning from my shoulders to my toes. I vowed to defeat the physical problems that attacked me. Determined, I reclaimed my "woman of iron" identity.

Conversations with loved ones varied little.

"How do you feel?" my sister asked.

"Exhausted and very pained, but I'll have to find a way to get myself to Macy's because they'll hold the new drapes on sale for me until tomorrow."

"It sounds as if those drapes are much more important than getting your rest."

There was that word "rest" again. I had heard it so many times when Mom was hospitalized with pneumonia, but she never stopped to rest once she got home. Whenever I heard her coughing, I told her to sit down and rest. The word sounded right, but it was non-operative.

In the months that passed after Dr. Barrett made the SLE diagnosis, stiff joints accompanied the pain. Currents of exhaustion traveled through my body. I kept up the daily ritual, getting up, teaching, correcting papers, meeting with students, writing articles, eating, and talking with friends, but my heart was not in it. Only the fear of losing my job and not having money to pay for healthcare kept me functioning.

I continued researching SLE. As frightening as most of the information read, I fixated on reports that showed some hope. About 4% of people might experience complete recovery from this chronic illness. With attention to the 4%, I attended a series of conferences at the Stanford Medical Center designed for women fully intent on "beating it." The language sounded strong and convincing, yet my goal was less about "beating the illness" than about trying to understand how it might manifest in me and to learn about possible treatments. The "beating the illness" slogan felt too violent for me to embrace. I wanted to learn what to expect of this condition. I knew that if I understood the anatomy of the illness, I would be less afraid. It seemed impossible to control an illness, but I did want to control my fear about the condition that was controlling me.

Most of the time, I rejected the readings that labeled my health condition as "acute" and "chronic." They felt pessimistic and permanent. I had no intention of amending the fast-paced life I led. This made it easier to disregard the labels associated with this autoimmune illness. From the onset of

SLE, I continued working as a full-time professor despite the distress signals from my body. I had too much work to do, and pain was not going to stand in the way. Illness was a sign of weakness. After all, personal achievements had taught me that the body existed to serve me.

In my steadfast, frenzied tempo at work, I ignored Dr. Barrett's cautions to "slow down." She told me, "The problem is complicated by your medical history, so now the drugs that we need to help you are failing us." However, my persistent complaints convinced her to escalate my medications. During one visit, she said, "I've done all I can to keep you going in a very fast-paced career and lifestyle. True, we're all caught in a mad pace, but you need to consider how you can get more rest." Is she serious? I wondered. She wants me to slow down even more? The crutches are taking care of that for me. By now I had reached a point of total exhaustion, unable to walk without a cane even around the house. But a new reality came home when Dr. Barrett insisted, "You are not taking responsibility for your part of healing. I'm going to put you on Lukeran to shut down your immune system and allow it to heal itself." It was a decisive moment. Up to this point, I hadn't been telling the truth to myself or to those around me.

Telling the truth about an illness means confronting the uncomfortable. At that point, I was not ready for that level of discomfort. Others I knew had made the leap. I knew this because when I became ill, some relationships changed—for the better, I would like to think. People felt more comfortable talking to me about their private ordeals with health than before. Tom, a university colleague, shared how his debilitating kidney illness had forced him and his wife to break through the fear of talking about illness. She had been reluctant to talk about his health. After Tom confronted his own fear, he told his wife, "I want to continue living as a whole person for as long as I'm alive. I don't want to think of myself as a broken person because of my kidney condition." Tom's wife understood his desire to talk openly and overcome the fear of the future.

Tom added, "I told her that no one knew what the future would bring, but I wanted us to talk about it all because even though the illness debilitated me physically, I didn't want it to debilitate our relationship."

Bravo for Tom. His words, "a whole person," inspired me. I applauded his courage to articulate his fear. Being a whole person sounded like a good idea, but for me it was still an abstraction. I was too busy with work and healthcare treatments to examine my relationships. While I reaped many coveted rewards and awards from working excessively, I noticed that I could no longer control the illness as I was accustomed to controlling the rest of my life. It was becoming clear that no matter how hard I worked, my body had limits. Physical endurance was central in obtaining the external awards and achievements I craved. Without it, I faced the unknown.

As Tom had felt during a time in his illness, I felt disconnected from my inner presence; denying that anything was wrong was my survival—or so I thought! Dr. Barrett referred me to a new internist, to neurologists, a cardiologist, a urologist, an optometrist, and a dermatologist to treat the various complications that were developing. I dragged myself to appointments with doctors and therapists, which consumed hours every day. But I did not ease my university teaching. I corrected midterm essays, prepared for lectures, edited journal articles, and read students' doctoral papers while waiting in offices and outpatient hospital rooms.

Work and Health Challenges

Over time, my work and healthcare worlds blended into one. When I tired of reading academic materials in doctors' waiting rooms, I turned to reading inspirational books. Marianne Williams, Clarissa Pinkola Estés, and Larry Dossey, among others, accompanied me as I looked for the word "hope" to distract me from the doctors' familiar and repetitive refrains: "There are complications, but we don't know why you're not responding to the medications." Their reports only made me dig in my heels, dropping the word "no" from my vocabulary.

I responded yes to everything. The result was a workaholic pace. It accomplished one thing: I felt in charge and productive though my body increasingly made me feel out of control. In reality, I was still in denial. How could a body require so much nurturing? Nothing in my academic or personal background had informed me that the body needed so much care. Whenever I had to see a doctor, I wanted just one thing: "Give me the strongest thing you have. I don't have time for this."

One thing I had to make time for was buying a different car. Driving a stick-shift strained my hips and shoulders. Using a clutch and gearshift exacerbated the debilitation and the joint and muscle burn. I had to buy a car with an automatic transmission. Mounting medical bills made a new car out of the question. A used one would have to do. My pre-owned automatic kept me on overdrive around town. The car represented a strong determination to keep my foot on the pedal—but it also deceived me into thinking that all was fine.

Invitations to universities across the country and abroad kept me in touch with groups that read my books. One group of anthropologists from the University of Granada invited me to speak in their summer series on international immigrant communities. Dr. Barrett and my family and friends insisted that I take it easy as much as possible to get strong enough to travel. I accomplished that.

The Laboratory of anthropology at the University of Granada, in Spain, invited me to lecture at their institute, where scholars from universities in Italy and Spain would also address issues of immigrants in their part of Europe. It sounded important enough. These were all issues that I had written about and had felt confident that I could teach. Then my body's new identity kicked in. Feelings of insecurity about the words I couldn't remember in English intensified with the prospect of lecturing in Spanish. I wrote out my lectures verbatim as I had done months earlier in university classes when my long and short-term memory lapsed. On the way to the airport, I complained to Eric, my partner, about the amount of work I had done to prepare for lecturing in Spain.

"You're making it too difficult for yourself," he said.

"I need to feel prepared."

"You're an expert in the field; why are you so preoccupied with writing out every word of your lectures?"

I looked out the window, wanting to scream with frustration. Words failed me. I couldn't explain that I had lost the language I needed for work. Now every word of my lectures had to be programmed, planned, and written. It was my way of staying in the academia game.

My lectures in Spain were totally successful; however, I quickly began to feel the physical strain of smoky trains, coffeehouses, long lectures, and endless conversations with students and colleagues from European universities. Exhausted, I got on a plane and headed for San Francisco.

Home again, I looked forward to starting the new quarter at the university, but I had barely enough strength to push open the heavy door to my office. With deep faith, I believed that my health problems would end if I did the "right" thing. Daily, I felt proud for taking responsibility through healthy nutrition, strengthening exercises, meditation, and prayer. But respite from the pain and complications was brief. I developed a bronchial infection, complete with fevers, fatigue, and burning joints and muscles. I resorted to using forearm crutches to get around.

On campus, getting to class required major orchestration; the university still refused to provide me shuttle service from my office to classes and other meetings. "You're not on our route," they explained. The university bureaucracy was not making this any easier. My forearm crutches would have to get me to the classroom—one slow step at a time; it was a painful thirty-minute walk.

At home, I was taking care to nap when I felt sleepy during the day. I usually fell asleep reading during that hour. Other times my favorite Laurindo Almeida classical guitar music relaxed me to sleep. Am I resting, I wondered?

Whether resting or working, emptiness became my constant companion. Is emptiness a feeling? No one answered. Somewhere I had misplaced Concha. She was lost.

Sunlight always boosted my spirits. One day, the birds chirped as I got ready to leave for a standing appointment with Dr. Barrett. The sun broke through the sheer curtains, inviting me to open them. It seemed so bright for a January day. The heater in my house still read eighty degrees, feeling barely warm. I hummed my way to the kitchen to prepare a standard yogurt and banana breakfast. With the radio in the background, I hobbled back to the bedroom, and on the NPR morning pro-gram I heard the programmer announce, "Thank you for joining us on this Wednesday, April 22." That's not possible, I thought. Something was wrong. In disbelief, I changed the station only to confirm that everyone was operating on a different calen-dar from mine. All of the months before had vanished from my mind. I could not account for anything I had done during those months, or how I now found myself in April, the previ-ous months a blank page. All my calendar entries were mean-ingless. I had no recall of the activities or any place I had been in the past three and a half months.

I felt hollow in mind and body, deceived by my strongest allies though they had kept me in control. Driving to Dr. Bar-rett's, I turned on a Carmen MacRae tape, but even she could not sing me out of the fog now shrouding my mind. I tried to describe to Dr. Barrett how I felt, but the most common words to describe the condition, as well as feelings, dates, and many people's names escaped me. I pointed to my wrists, "They've–they've been quite pained lately."

"Your wrists, you mean?"

"Yes, wrists, wrists," I repeated.

Trying to discern meaning from my choppy information, Dr. Barrett asked, "Are you having some problems focusing?"

I told her about the months of memory loss that had caught up with me that very morning. She was compassionate and reassured me that she would do everything possible to help me. After examining and questioning me, she referred me to Dr. Sanders, a neurologist, for a complete assessment.

More MRI tests and spinal taps. I called my friend Berta to bare my soul: "Tests are inconclusive, but the neurologist suspects some complications. Oh God, here come more bills.

Hope we can get to the bottom of this. I am totally broke and my memory is failing.

In her usual supportive way Berta said, "What a life!" Then she added, "Maybe you won't remember it!" We laughed. I was losing recall, but family and friends' laughter kept me going.

A month later, I had an appointment with the neurologist. I wanted to impress Dr. Sanders by acting physically stronger and more mentally alert than I really was. She followed me out the door as I left her office, watching every step. Standing at the car door, I dug into my purse for the keys. No luck. Dr. Sanders asked, "Can I help you?"

"I might have left my keys in your office."

"Wait here, I'll check."

I continued searching for them, and finally emptied my purse on top of the car. Dr. Sanders returned to say that she hadn't found the keys. I shoved everything back into my purse and again walked to the driver's door. Feeling rather frazzled, I peered through the window. From the door to her building, Dr. Sanders called, "Are they inside the car?"

"Yes, I see them." They were dangling from the ignition, and the radio was on. Foolish doesn't begin to describe how I felt. So much for my facade. Dr. Sanders spent the next half-hour helping me get the keys out of the car.

Losing track of time, destinations, concepts, and friendly faces forced me to keep a daily journal, which I carried everywhere. The memory loss was not imaginary; the journal notes confirmed my suspicions that frequent lapses were occurring, chunks of time vanishing. Doctors explained that people with chronic autoimmune illnesses experience memory loss differently. In my case, it sneaked up on me insidiously.

At times, we all have selective memory, but forgetting chunks of one's life events produces devastating confusion and fear. Facts, names, dates, and ideas leaked out of my memory bank until I felt blank. My connection with my childhood, family, and past experience was as foreign as my present. Vainly, I tried to trivialize each memory loss that occurred, but the effort of remembering what to do when I entered my classroom at the university was a strange odyssey.

In the mornings, handfuls of hair on my pillow signaled another stage of this condition. Fortunately, the curly hair look was fashionable. On a good day, I also covered the huge bald spots with hair crayons. These were quite different from the box of twenty-four brightly colored crayons I recalled using in elementary school. "Your hair loss is probably due to the lupus," said Dr. Barrett.

Admittedly, when I stopped to think about it, I felt grateful for little things I was still able to do. Without this condition, I wouldn't appreciate that brushing my teeth and combing my hair involve the back, shoulders, biceps, forearms, wrists, and hands. These were actions and motions that were automatic before. How unconscious we are of our bodies! Maybe it's a good thing. We'd never accomplish much if we had to calculate every movement in our day. Now my world was choreographed in exactly that way.

Insisting on maintaining the image of a professor in charge of her career, I dressed and looked the part, but what stared back at me in the mirror was an ugly body that I could not control. This illness thrust me out there in public. It was embarrassing for someone who thrived on privacy.

As much as people reassured me about my appearance, I still feared looking ill with every hair that fell. Soon, face make-up became my public mask to deflect attention from the straggly few strands of hair and the bruised-looking face that was now a perfectly round moon shape. Eric said, "Don't put on that messy make-up. You look fine without it. Natural is best." "You always look so sharp," people assured me. Sincere as the compliments sounded, I rejected them, imagining that people were merely trying to make me feel better.

The irony of it all! For years, my profession as a researcher had placed me in the middle of people's real-life dramas. Now the tables were turned. I became the subject of a medical puzzle with more questions than answers. I sank deeper into feelings of powerlessness. Every visit to the rheumatologist forced me to write down my complaints so that I could get the words out while in her office: "There's relentless pain in every joint — tender to the touch, all over my body. My muscles are so weak that it hurts to breathe. I feel as though I've sprinted five miles and can't catch my breath. I don't even want to talk."

Glancing up from her notes Dr. Barrett asked, "If you rest, can you regain your breath?"

"Not completely. All day long I'm so exhausted that I feel faint. It frightens me and interferes with my work." She wrote ferociously on the sheet that would go into my file.

Much like those early years of learning English when I was suddenly in a new culture and didn't understand the language, once again I doubted my ability to make myself understood. Regardless of how much Dr. Barrett and I talked, there seemed to be much more information that I needed, but so often I didn't even know what questions to ask. Here I was, a university professor, tongue-tied in doctors' offices, unable to describe the frightening condition that impaired me physically and now linguistically.

Should I lie down and stay in bed until I don't feel fatigue? What can I do that I'm not already doing when I almost faint with fatigue?

Dr. Barrett offered a comment: "It sounds as if the swings in your energy level are still extreme."

"My legs buckle under my depleted body, which feels like a lead weight."

Friends who knew me well expected an update on my medical exams and progress. Every time I saw them, they pitched question after question.

"Do the tests show you're improving?"

"Are you doing all you can to help yourself?"

The one question I feared asking was, "Is this now the new normal for me? Is this the best I can expect in the way of improvement?"

An insecure smile hid the pain and shielded me from unwanted questions. If I appeared cheerful, I could often deflect the expected inquiries. Besides, frowning requires more muscles. Often I just wanted to protect people from feeling concerned about my situation. The more concerned they were, the more questions they asked. Having answers to every question was part of my need to remain in control. Now I wonder why I couldn't just answer truthfully, "I don't know!" I had run out of answers that would satisfy my friends and me.

At night, Berta's call was a chance for me to release. She got an earful.

"I hate it when people ask me how I'm feeling."

"They care about you."

"I know, but I can't keep explaining so much. It tires me."

"The people who care about you feel powerless. They want to know how to help."

Berta had come about this wisdom when her son Gavin had cancer while a student at UC Santa Barbara. I had known Gavin since he was a five-year-old. He was a dear friend. During his struggle with cancer, we shared readings on healing. He went on to redirect his life and gain the physical and inner strength to become his own person. Years later, Gavin was killed in a car accident. Just before his death, Gavin wrote that the year prior to discovering he had cancer, he had been floundering and feeling empty in his life. By healing the cancer, he had found his true strength. Thereafter he made personal relationships his primary focus in life. He spoke through Berta's voice, urging me to harness the love of those around me. Was it possible that I was shutting out my body and that it was in turn shouting out at me, telling me something that I didn't want to hear? I had been so concerned with not having words to stay in the world I knew. Was my body trying to tell me to live differently? The question was out there. I feared the answer, since I had no clue as to what "different" would look like. And I had no energy to contemplate it.

In defiance of my body's condition, I continued to teach full-time at the university and attend meetings on campus. I also traveled to research sites in Southern California, Alaska, and Mexico, and presented keynote addresses at human development symposia at Cornell University, the University of Cincinnati, and UCLA. My ego always seemed to find reasons for accepting.

One time the UCLA School of Management invited me to lecture about my research on empowering communities and forging partnerships between families, schools, and businesses.

I felt committed to supporting this school-reform effort spear-headed by UCLA. By the time the participants arrived at the hall, I felt pained and fatigued. When I began speaking, the audi-ence couldn't hear me. The performance skills so familiar to me for many years failed me. The technicians had to place four microphones close to my face so that the audience of almost 1000 people could hear. Despite the ordeal, audiences appreci-ated the presentation. There it was — the reason for persisting in my work. It rewarded me. Without an identity more mean-ingful than the body, I had to hang on, fearing that I would have no identity if my body didn't perform as before.

One question I could always count on from Dr. Barrett was "Are you getting enough rest?"

"Yes," I always answered, "I am." But this wasn't the case.

Rest!

Rest!

Rest!

How can I get any work done? Days crammed with appoint-ments — where's the time? And if I stop to rest I'll focus on illness and it becomes real! The other problem was that I remained clueless as to the meaning of the word "rest." What do people do when they rest? Read a book? Friends said that they rested by reading books. I'll read mysteries, I thought. Yes, a book. Or, I could sit down. Just sit? What a waste of time! Maybe ten minutes will suffice if done right. Maybe it is nothingness — like meditation — just paying attention to my breath.

After leaving the rheumatologist's office, I wondered why I hadn't told her that I really didn't know what she meant by "rest." I recalled from childhood how my parents used to say that an idle person was a lazy person. In all the years I lived with them, I never recalled seeing either of my parents sitting or resting. I certainly never wanted people to think I was lazy. I had shaped a lifestyle around that very belief. The concept of rest remained foreign to me.

Dr. Barrett suggested at least an hour of bed rest daily. "It's mandatory," she insisted. "And if you have to go to campus, you should increase your rest on the days before and after."

"Okay," I responded. Now I had a fixed time schedule to guide me, if I could get past the embarrassment of asking what one did while resting. Enough ambiguity for now! I took a chance that I could clarify what I needed to know to help myself.

"What should I do when I rest? Sleep?" I asked Dr. Barrett.

"Sleep if you need to, but it's not necessary. You have to listen to what your body needs. "But," Dr. Barrett underscored, "your immune system does need to rest."

More ambiguity. I had learned an important feature of this phenomenon called rest, but it was no easier to activate it. What does it mean to "listen to what your body needs"? I was listening, and all I heard was flaming screams! That's why I was here in a doctor's office trying to get answers. I couldn't hear anything but a raw cry. How does one listen to a body? I yelled in silence in my journal. What can rest mean?

Repose?

Relax?

Calm down?

Be tranquil?

Be peaceful?

Be still?

Be quiet?

I had two words to describe the state of my body: acute and chronic. Acute is synonymous with fierce, intense, profound, severe, and relentless. Chronic, on the other hand, means constant, persistent, continuous, unrelenting, consistent, and unflagging. To be sure, these two adjectives were part of the language that I feared defined the situation as permanent.

I now know that in our country's medical system, what we don't know can hurt us. When you have an incurable illness, no one can tell you what to expect, how to conduct your daily life, how to deal with relapses, how to accept constant pain, and how to look good when you feel destroyed. To become active participants in our healthcare we need language that gives us access to information that empowers us to make choices on our behalf. Since doctors don't always tell us what we need to know because they're not always certain, we need to listen to the healer within that speaks for us.

We need to educate ourselves. It is imperative that we become accountable and proactive in healing our lives. Before being diagnosed with SLE, I had no idea what it meant to heal one's life, and the more I focused on getting well the more stressed I felt. I had to find a different way to live. I longed to return to that healthy and tranquil pace I walked in Alaska.

At home in California, I lived in another type of silence—denial. Insisting that life continue as before kept me stuck in the belief that my body was there to achieve my goals. My body, however, was exhausted from the daily fast track. I was divided: one part insisted on a fast pace, the other craved a slow and healing stride. The two lived in opposition to one another. Although work was quite intense, it alone was not the problem; placing work first relegated my health to a position of lower priority. All the while, the voiceless part of me screamed through the pain, wanting to take charge.

CHAPTER 5

Demystifying Labels

Illness has a built-in compass; through it,
we can discover who we really are....

Gradually, I learned to surrender to rest. Resting, I faced my aching body and pained heart that wanted to move forward, out of the disabled condition. The word "disabled" made me cringe. Too many symbols identified me as belonging in the "disabled" world. As reminders, there were canes, forearm crutches, medical treatments, and a blue placard hanging on my rearview mirror. My career vitae, on the other had, identified me as a very able person. After all, I was a professor at the University of California. I had earned prestigious awards for research. Was it possible that I lived in two worlds? Could one be able and disabled at the same time?

These questions jarred me to reject the word "disabled" as I read and studied how society labels us in convenient categories. The need for such labels is not all bad. Oftentimes, funds for services to specific populations are based on their needs for treatment and education. Thus, describing people's medical condition is necessary. *Who determines the label applied to us? Who decides that I am physically disabled?* I asked myself. While my body said, "I am disabled," my heart said, "I am able, despite my body's condition."

During my life, I had crossed many borders—geographic, linguistic, social, and cultural. Now, moving between the "able" and "disabled" borders kept me questioning what my body could do and not do and kept me wondering who was judging.

In my dreams, my former able-bodied identity would visit. I ran or danced blissfully. Walking onto an elegantly decorated dance floor where a faceless crowd stood and talked, I didn't want to be there until I heard the band begin to play. Suddenly, I was in my dashing partner's arms, ballroom dancing a glamorous waltz, then a spirited mambo. I was free. This was the Concha I knew. But as early daylight entered my room, I immediately felt abandoned in the cold, silent morning. A wave of sadness shifted my consciousness as I slipped into the pain-saturated body that awakened me. Images of my healthy body lingered as I sat up for meditation. Following such dreams, I tearfully poised myself at the edge of the bed, grabbed the chair, and pressed against the wall to balance myself. Recalling the dream of twisting and turning on the dance floor put a smile on my face. Hope began the day.

The word "compromised" was popular with doctors. I knew the meaning of the word, but not in this context. They all asked, "How compromised are you?"

"Compromised?" I asked. "I continue getting lung infections; my digestive system is on fire and I have recurring spasms; my legs are cold and numb from the knees down, and they're very weak; the stinging, burning joint pain is unbearable. I think that's the skeletal system, but I'm not sure; my eyes are blurry a lot of the time; and all my muscles burn and are weak; oh yes, my hair keeps falling out. I don't know why."

"Anything else? Dr. Barrett asked.

"Isn't that enough?"

"It must be hard."

"I don't care how hard it is. I just want it to end."

Every medical exam meant an avalanche of doctors' questions, pushing me deeper into the category of disabled.

How does it feel if I squeeze here?

What kind of pain?

How about here?

What if I raise this arm?

What about this hip?

What kind of pain does that produce?

Let's see you raise your leg on your own, can you do it?

How does that feel?

How far can you raise it from here? Does that hurt? How much? How does it feel?

Can you push against my hand?

Can we reproduce that pain if I apply pressure here?

If I squeeze your knee, does it hurt?

How about your wrist; if you turn it, what happens?

When you raise your arm, does that produce pain?

Every examination revealed a life in constant change. I was unable to take long drives on Sunday afternoons; unable to sit up and write until 3:00 in the morning; unable to enjoy long chats on the phone with friends because my breath waned.

Are you working? How much?

Are you driving your car? How far?

Do you do housework? What kind?

Can you push a vacuum cleaner? How long?

What kind of help do you have at home?

Do you have a support system?

The effort to respond intensified my exhaustion and pain. And this was not enough. Dr. Barrett wanted a precise description of the pain. I paused, repeating the word over and over in my mind. Again, I was eight years old, wearing uncomfortable, oversized black-and-white oxford shoes that blistered my ankles, staring into the teacher's disapproving face. I explained to her in what was a foreign language to me that I didn't know the word that matched the picture in the book. In Dr. Barrett's office, I ached for words to fill the blanks of her quiz in this new language of disability that I resented learning. Only one word came to mind to describe the pain: horrible.

She looked at me from behind her small reading glasses. "Horrible?"

Is it pain if my arms feel thick and heavy even when they aren't moving? I'm confused—I don't know what I think anymore! I can't feel hips! They don't move when I walk. Why won't my legs bend? Is it pain if you don't feel it and can't use it? In my mind, I scrolled down a picture thesaurus of how pain engulfed my body.

PAIN!

Burning. Stinging. Throbbing. Pinching. Aching.

Stabbing. Shooting. Tremor. Pang. Spasm.

Intense. Heavy. Tender. Thick. Severe.

Unbearable. Like hot salsa running through my veins. Burning—yes that's it! But it's not that simple. "What degree?" the doctor wants to know.

I knew this pain was like a third-degree burn. A memory of ten-year-old Concha flashed before me. It was a Saturday afternoon and I was responsible for cooking the rice for lunch. I lifted the lid from the pot when the rice was boiling, and a burst of steam escaped and burnt my thumb so raw that the skin fell off. The doctors who bandaged it at the emergency room said it was a third-degree burn.

The old saying, "necessity is the mother of invention," governed my adult life with pain. I found ways to simplify my household routines. In the kitchen, making one-dish meals saved energy in preparing and cleaning up. One night I was trying to bake red snapper in the oven, and as I reached in for the Pyrex pan, I felt a hot spot near my wrist. The sizzle I heard was not the snapper. It was my skin. The burn had created a hole about a quarter inch wide and deep enough to show white tissue. I put ice, Polysporin ointment, and a Band-Aid on it. A week later, I found myself in the emergency room to deal with a respiratory complication. The attending doctor asked why I had a Band-Aid on my wrist. I showed him the burn and he asked me, "Does it hurt?"

"Not any more than the rest of my body."

"I'm concerned that it still looks raw."

"It's been that way."

"That's a third-degree burn you've got there. It must hurt."

"Not any more than the rest of me," I repeated.

More exhausting than the pain was the dread of my new identity as a disabled person. I resisted the "disabled" label that haunted me, shaking my confidence and belief that I had any abilities left.

At home, I wondered if Eric or my family and friends tired of me complaining about pain. Although family members called frequently, I wondered whether friends hesitated to invite me out because I tired so easily. Did colleagues at the university see me as less capable than the productive person I had always been?

Work demands made me wonder if my body could keep up with the day-to-day pressures of the profession. The six-hour drive down to my research site in southern California afforded me plenty of time to contemplate my concerns. Singing along with oldies on the radio, I appreciated how my work fed the researcher, the scholar, and the advocate in me who wanted to improve the world by working with communities to empower themselves through literacy. When I was nourished by these thoughts, having to drive long distances, attend meetings, and collect interviews all in the span of thirty-six hours seemed less of a grind.

As a researcher, I've been privileged to work with many wonderfully dynamic communities. Carpinteria, a small town twenty minutes south of Santa Barbara, is one. In this community of five schools, Latino and white families lived across the freeway from each other. However, children from both sides of town met up in the schools. My collaboration as a researcher and facilitator with the families in Carpinteria gave me entrance to the complexities of their lives. I saw the painful aspects that many do not see. The families in Carpinteria lived with joblessness, alcohol abuse, teen pregnancy, infidelity, and catastrophic illness, as well as the heartbreak of their children's academic underachievement, general stress, and burnout. Still, they rallied and answered the call to come forth and get involved.

I observed many of these families' home and community literacy practices. As they learned more about each other, they realized that they were not alone. They shared common concerns, especially about their children's education. I met with them to share my observations. We gathered frequently to talk about the issues facing them — and that was the beginning of a new conversation.

In Carpinteria, my work and my life in this pained body over-lapped. This community's actions for social change became an inspiration. They confronted their perceived limitations, took action in uncomfortable ways to change their conditions in life, and formed a strong collective by teaching and support-ing one another to learn a new culture and language so that they could help their children in their schooling.

I observed how a small group of seven parents in Carpin-teria united to break the cycle of social and cultural barriers. They organized themselves into a district-wide group for the purpose of supporting other parents in the community. Col-lectively, these parents provided each other a supportive learn-ing environment! Through collective reflection, they turned their crises into opportunities to learn, and discovered their strengths. From each other they realized the importance of being role models for their children by taking English classes and completing their high school education. Some even went on to community college for training in nursing and preschool teaching. They wanted to show their children how important it was to always keep learning. In effect, these parents empow-ered themselves.

In the year that followed, this small group expanded to include all the Latino families in all of the Carpinteria schools. They continued transforming themselves through common language and shared history. The leaders worked with the principals and teachers in each school to organize the parents.

The first parent meeting at an elementary school brought out over a hundred Spanish-speaking parents. In the school audi-torium on a Friday evening, the parent leaders presented the group's goals and invited those present to join them by orga-nizing a local parent group in that school. People were quick to state their limitations: Too little time, no child-care, don't know what to say at meetings, and other excuses for not getting involved. But a most encouraging comment came from Mr. Sosa, one of the men leading the meeting. He said (my translation from Spanish):

> No one up here has any experience with schools or with forming organizations. Our only common experience is parenthood as Spanish-speaking families in Carpinteria. We come here tonight to ask you to help us. Together we can learn from each other. We can build a support system for our children through our families. There is no experience necessary—only willingness to act on behalf of our children.

This time, people couldn't raise their hands fast enough to join in. Within minutes, there were enough volunteers to form a school-site committee.

Parents and educators collaborated to shape strong learning opportunities for all students. Their collective journey led them to new visions, demonstrating resilience while forming a new sense of self. The people in Carpinteria built bridges to travel out and learn from each other, and return home with a deeper sense of self.

Anthropologist Mary Catherine Bateson, daughter of renowned anthropologists Margaret Mead and Gregory Bateson, comments in her book *Peripheral Visions*, "In all, learning is change, becoming slightly or profoundly different. But learning is welcome when it affirms a continuing sense of self."[3]

It was because these people were growing and learning more about themselves that their spiral of empowerment kept expanding. I couldn't help thinking about myself: was I learning and growing through my situation? I learned a great deal from this community.

At one meeting, Mrs. Rojas, who became the group's first president, spoke to parents about their worthiness: that of caring for their children, speaking a beautiful language, and sharing important world views with them. She added that they, as parents, transmitted their cultural values and history to their children. Mrs. Rojas felt strongly that Latinos should organize because, as she put it, "*Venemos porque podemos, no a ver si podemos.*" ("We've come here because we can, not to see if we can.") This became the quintessential motto of the parent group. They acknowledged their power, which enabled them to confront their deficit behaviors.

Those words were forever etched in my mind. These families understood that they could not let others' perceptions of their deficits hold them back. They wanted to proceed from a position of strength. Their energy was contagious. Transcending one's limitations opens the door to countless possibilities, even if we don't know what lies ahead.

I don't believe that one needs a crisis to discover one's power. Rather, I believe that the process of empowerment begins at any point and moves forward without end. It is an ongoing process in perpetual motion. Building on knowledge we already have, the spiral grows from there, engaging more people along the way. Imagine a tornado picking up momentum as it travels—except that in this case, its outcome is not destruction. Rather, it creates cycles of new knowledge while building stronger relationships.

For the parent leaders, reaching others by sharing their personal experience connected them to each other and to the educators who taught their children. Mary Catherine Bateson reinforces that point: "When we struggle to respond to the unpredictable and unfamiliar, learning new skills transmutes discomfort and bewilderment into valuable information."

Turning vulnerabilities into strengths, the parent leadership group reached out to every school. Their power base grew, one school at a time.

This Carpinteria group's total commitment to their children impressed me in countless ways. Every time we conversed about the growth they had experienced since we began working together as a collective, I saw the transformative power of facing obstacles when we obtain support by joining with others. During one conversation, parents revealed to each other that they had learned how their power resided with them. Mr. Gomez summarized the group spirit of empowerment. (Translated from Spanish: "The reality is that we are very different people than we were when we first met.") Mrs. Chavez added: "The Spanish-speaking Latino community now has a voice, which is legitimate and heard. In our families, we have more communication between our children and ourselves as parents. And we participate more directly in our children's schooling."

On crutches, I watched these families unite in community to transform the perceived cultural deficit labels that they and others had imposed on them. They looked within and to each other and discovered their strengths in community. I, too, could learn to go beyond the label of disabled to focus on the strong part of me.

Stretching Beyond Comfort

Carpinteria families reminded me that I belonged not only to one loving community but to many. Back in the Bay Area, I turned to family and friends for comfort after receiving news from the neurologist. "Your physical weakness seems to be increasing. This concerns me. We can't risk a fall. I'm prescribing a power wheelchair to assist you."

Images of sitting in a wheelchair shrunk my world to minuscule size. Since this illness began, whenever I appeared in my dreams, I walked, ran, or danced freely. Now the prospect of using a wheelchair became all too real. One night my fears took the form of a convincing nightmare. A large figure I couldn't discern pushed me into a wheelchair and told me I could not get out of it. After I made futile efforts to stand, the chair, with me in it, rolled out of control down an empty dark corridor. I couldn't see where it was going, and though I cried out for help, my screams went unheard. Panic jolted me awake.

Nothing had changed. I felt as empty as the corridor in my dream. I wanted so much to believe what Buddhists say about emptiness, that emptiness in life is necessary in order to see our connection to the rest of the universe. Unfortunately, my mind wasn't there yet, but I tried to hold on to the idea that we are not empty if we're connected to the universe.

Dr. Sanders prescribed a power wheelchair because I had been increasingly losing mobility in my arms and legs. I still resisted the idea of using the chair. As far as I was concerned, the forearm crutches I used were sufficient support. I had learned to walk, deliberately, counting every step from one end of the room to another.

Expecting a miraculous recovery overnight, I held on to the wheelchair prescription. Finally, I relented. The salesman rang my doorbell. He wore a smile and was dressed in a dark-green jumpsuit. "Ms. Delgado," he said, "I've brought a model with me so that you can see how you feel sitting in it. We'll order it in any color you want."

"Teal is fine."

Surprisingly, sitting in the wheelchair felt very comfortable. If only I could change my mind about riding around in it. Could I get past the fear that my condition would become permanent if I used it? Feeling less physical pain while sitting in the wheelchair made me realize that I had to get practical. Talks with the wise inner voice convinced me that I could conserve energy by using the wheelchair around the office, leaving me more strength to enjoy recreation. The self-imposed stigma disappeared. In fact, I felt stronger about myself as a person. Increasingly, I was able to suspend judgment against myself whenever my health declined.

People with a chronic illness talk about how difficult it is for loved ones to be constantly "on standby." I required a handful of people to stand by, not knowing when I might call on them to assist me. People may truly want to help, but it's difficult for caretakers who can never know when the "need" will end—worse yet, if it's a permanent ordeal! My loved ones felt equally frustrated by not knowing how to help me get well. Fearing that I was imposing on others made me more reluctant to call on anyone when I was alone during hard times.

Luis, my spiritual mentor, always insisted that I call him at any hour of the day or night. He encouraged me to stretch beyond my limitations. "You need to reach out and ask for help when you need it. We're not in this world to do it alone. The only way to heal your belief that you have to take care of yourself is by reaching out." I heard Luis. Still, I hesitated before reaching out, even if loved ones expected me to call on them.

A giant step for me was allowing my pastor, Ken, to organize a list of people from the congregation. They were my "helping hands." I updated the list continuously as people's schedules changed. That list, kept near the phone, reminded me that I was a part of a supportive community.

Work did not let up. It intensified the pain, yet distracted me from worrying about it. A daily regimen of strengthening exercises at home pushed me through the pain. Dr. Barrett suggested, "You need to do more hydrotherapy exercises. In the pool you don't put as much pressure on your knees."

"Pools are too cold for me."

"Go to the heated pool for seniors and the disabled. Sign up with the Arthritis Foundation."

The Berkeley High School pool was a perfect ninety degrees. I couldn't wait for late afternoons, when I pushed open the giant, heavy door. Inside the building, the Olympic-size pool occupied all but the narrow walkways around it. The lifeguards greeted all of us by our first names. The lifeguard at the pool took the towel bag hanging on my shoulder and accompanied me to the steps leading into the pool. Outside the pool, people differed in their ability to walk, sit, limp, talk, and use forearm crutches, wheelchairs, and braces. Some had full limbs but suffered with ailments that were not apparent. Others were paraplegic or quadriplegic. Some walked erect but were blind. For me, it took fifteen minutes to walk from the front door to the locker room so I could remove my jogging suit.

Inside the pool, we were equal. Water is very forgiving. Most of us stayed afloat on our own. A few came to the pool with caregivers who guided around the floating devices. For over an hour, I did the backstroke and alternated with a cross-country skiing motion in the deep end, with a floater belt around my waist, strengthening my cardiovascular system.

Performing hydrotherapy exercises, I was reminded of the one-eyed man in the valley of the blind. In past years, I had assigned one of my classes to read *The Country of the Blind* by H. G. Wells. The story is about a community whose residents had been blind for fourteen generations and had been cut off from the entire sighted world. Names for all the things that people could see had faded and changed. They created a new culture, a new language with new imagination through other senses that grew more sensitive. A partially sighted man who was lost found himself in the country of the blind. He believed that he was superior to them because he could see. In time, he learned to appreciate their values, as they convinced him that their lives were complete without sight. I had come so far as to understand how I looked and moved like the people in the pool.

Before, I had thought of disabled people as "unable to do." That is not the case. The pool community opened my eyes to a new dimension of physical ability—that we are more than our physical body. Luis reinforced this every time we talked, but until I began using the pool, I didn't really grasp what he meant. The courage displayed by everyone I met at the pool inspired me. Everyone there had some form of disability, no matter how normal some bodies looked. I came face to face with my own resistance to seeing myself as a disabled person. The panic I felt about acknowledging my disability rose from a fear that if I accepted this label, it might become permanent. But in the pool, I learned that the label "disabled" didn't mean "limited."

"In the disabled community, we like to think of ourselves as people with diverse abilities," said Jesse, who used the pool.

"Diverse abilities?" questioned Berta. "What's that, some kind of New-Age concept?"

"No. It describes people by what they're capable of doing as opposed to how they're restricted."

"Good sense."

Appreciating myself where I was became significant in the healing process. Still, the idea that disabled meant having diverse abilities took awhile to accept. Ann, a physical therapist, assisted me in and out of the pool. She carefully observed my every movement, then commented, "You need to walk more slowly so that you're able to balance better and prevent a fall." She did everything to persuade me to stop carrying my towels and toiletries in a heavy shoulder bag. "Get yourself a bag on wheels. You shouldn't carry any weight on your arms or shoulders."

"I don't need a new bag. I'll be all right."

My reaction to Ann was evidence that I still resisted the disabled label. She finally convinced me, noting, "You know, 80% of Americans suffer from back problems, and none of those folks should carry heavy things because it stresses their troubled areas. Do this: get a bag with wheels for now, and if you're inclined to carry big bags on your shoulder, when you get well, you can carry them then." Residual resistance to being disabled made me reluctant, but Ann won me over as I adjusted my thinking. I soon acquiesced and bought a bag on casters. Everyone should take better care to walk more slowly so that they won't fall, and certainly, no one should carry heavy bags.

An invitation to lecture in Mexico provided another opportunity to reach out for support and to feel comfortable traveling as a disabled person in a wheelchair. I was invited to speak to the National Association of Educational Research in Mexico City. My hosts were apprised of my health difficulty and promised me good care. I had every reason to trust them. But friends were concerned. Yoli asked, "Are you sure that you can take this trip by yourself?"

"I've always traveled by myself. It'll be all right."

"Why don't you let me accompany you?"

"You have to work."

"I can afford a few days' leave to travel with you."

After the five-hour flight, a handsome man with black wavy hair and a disarming smile greeted us in Mexico City. He was assigned to be my personal chauffeur for the week. After Yoli and I arrived at the hotel, I willingly surrendered, exhausted, to the inviting bed.

Refreshed after a nap, I stood looking out the window of our hotel room, recalling my early days growing up in Chihuahua. Braided lights of red, green, and white, the colors of the Mexican flag, decorated buildings and plazas in honor of the National Independence Day festivities, which had begun on September 16, four days before. From our lovely hotel overlooking the *zocalo* (town square), I could see the Indian vendors who sat on the sidewalks to sell their wares.

Cobblestone sidewalks are unfriendly to wheelchairs. Moving me from the car to a building took three people to carry the wheelchair up the flights of stairs. Yes, there were wheelchair ramps, but they were built in impractical places leading to the back of the building where there was no entrance. I understood, firsthand, why I never saw a wheelchair in Mexico. What I did see was a vendor with one leg hobble down a street, carrying a load of ceramic dishes on his back to sell. A woman with one arm carried a baby wrapped around her upper body with a long *rebozo* (shawl). A young girl clung to her skirt, and a slightly older boy walked beside her, one hand holding his sister's hand, the other holding a bag of groceries.

On our flight home, I looked out the window and thought of the many people like me who would never have the comfort of a wheelchair when they needed it. I leaned over to Yoli and said, "The next time I complain about pain, please remind me about the people on canes navigating the cobblestone streets in Mexico." I totally appreciated the wheelchair ramps in the US. For all the conveniences available to disabled people, however, I knew that I would never be able to get along without the support of a loving community to remind me how "able" I really was.

CHAPTER 6

Embracing Miracles

Miracles are not things we wish for;
they are inspired by our freedom from fear.

From the day we met there was no hiding from Luis. He cut to the chase faster than anyone I knew. I was a professor at UC Santa Barbara when I met Luis, a middle-aged man who stood almost eye to eye with me. Although fair in complexion, his facial features revealed his Peruvian ethnicity. His willingness to listen to me made time spent with him healing in every way. He looked straight into my eyes, and said in deep Peruvian accent, "Tell me what's happening with you." His gift for getting to the heart of the problem with such clarity was amazing. At times, I resented his knowing me so well, but I appreciated the opportunity he provided to unravel my inner conflicts.

Luis was a minister in the Church of Religious Science who also taught meditation classes. In conversation, we learned that we shared a love of culture, music, poetry, and food. By the end of the first course I took with Luis, he and his wife, Patty, who was also a minister, became my good friends. They both encouraged and influenced me to pursue more contemplative study. From that point on, I enjoyed many of Luis's lectures and seminars on spirituality.

During the early years of my struggle with lupus, I relied on Luis to help me understand my condition with a fresh perspective. Talking with him helped me find the strength I needed. Luis based his approach to healing on the study and practice of psycho-spiritual integration. The idea was that healing occurred when one connected the body's immune system with one's emotions and spirituality. This was easier when I was home and could slow down, putting work aside for at least awhile.

I called on Luis for support. His refreshing optimism and profound insights always encouraged me. Yet, his bright outlook threatened my compulsive work habits. He took every opportunity to suggest, "You need to quit working and focus strictly on resting and actively working on your healing."

"Can't I hear my inner spirit while working?" I asked.

"You have competing priorities. You're driving your body in order to do your work. That's not healing."

One ear heard Luis's good intentions, while the other went deaf. It was easier for me to blame my excessive lifestyle for the persistent condition and recurring relapses than it was to confront the reality of the health tragedy that I didn't understand and couldn't control. To Luis, however, healing was closer than any doctor; my healer was within. I had trusted only my mental and physical strength. Luis was teaching me to see things from a different perspective, a different belief system. I was learning how to take care of myself. This meant making choices about cutting back on work, which I didn't want to do. Rethinking one's beliefs requires enormous energy. I wasn't sure I had the energy to make such major changes in my thinking. Changing medications or hydrotherapy pools seemed easier. Luis reassured me that he would support me through it. Before our conversation ended, I was convinced that new opportunities for healing were possible.

Stripped of all the assets that I believed made me worthy, a strong body and sharp mind, I feared what lay ahead. What might happen if I let go and stopped trying to control my circumstances? I wanted to return to my childhood days of innocent faith when things seemed safe, but also to practice what I already knew intellectually. Maybe spiritual readings from *A Course in Miracles*, which Luis suggested, would anchor me. Translating from abstract to habit called for a sage like Luis. Through our friendship, he taught me how to make spirituality come alive in daily life.

Luis was the ideal spiritual teacher, given his knowledge of metaphysics, psychology, philosophy, literature, and life. He taught me how to listen to my body's needs, that meditation and resting was part of spirituality, part of living consciously in the present. The one point of comparison that I had was in academia. In that world, one needs a good theory to provide a clear perspective and explain the bigger picture. I noticed that all the medical, physical, and nutritional therapies I experimented with had a specific set of beliefs designed to address only a small area of my problem. This became clear when one day I read the literature about one expensive vitamin-tonic supplement I drank. As effective as it was in boosting my physical energy during the day, I was clueless why other areas of my health weren't improving.

For the bigger picture, I relied more and more on readings from *A Course in Miracles* and the notions of "connectedness" and "oneness." Although too ethereal for me to grasp at times, these ideas piqued my interest. That I kept reading even when it didn't make sense to me was healing in itself. This meant that I could bypass the analytical aspect and sit with the meaning of the message. Was this the inner teacher in me that Luis wanted me to hear? Listening to that inner voice became easier when Luis incorporated a breathing meditation into my healing work with him. He explained that the deep-breathing work, which he supervised, helped me to safely confront feelings buried in my body. Consequently, when the immune system releases the pent-up stress, the system heals.

"Turn and face the beast," Luis instructed me. "That's the way to heal the immune system—you can't run from it anymore. You'll find that what looks like the beast is just another part of you that begs to be integrated into your being." Getting around on crutches was difficult enough, and traveling to Luis's office in Kern County almost weekly was in itself a feat! He lived an hour's flight away, and on Saturdays there was only one flight there. A friend drove me to San Francisco airport to get on a small shuttle plane.

Other times I dodged morning commute traffic to the airport, parked the car in the handicapped space by the elevators, grabbed my forearm crutches, stepped onto the elevator, and walked breathlessly past three ticket counters to board a 9:30 a.m. flight on a twelve-passenger express plane. Weathering the delays, I would arrive at Luis's just before noon. He always met me at the airport.

After our coffee chat, Luis and I went to his office, where we worked for two or three hours. Even before we began talking, I felt safe. It was as if I had already found the tranquillity. Luis and I sat on comfortable chairs facing each other. "How are you doing physically?" Luis began.

"Most of the time, I feel awful."

"That's got to be tough."

"Luis, I've been meditating and learning to pray differently, and the bodily discomfort and compounding infections persist."

"Well, you're still placing emphasis on the outer world."

"Okay, tell me what that means. I'm ready to listen."

"It means that you can't change what's outside of you."

"That's what I've been trying to do with meditation and prayer."

"That's fine. Now our work together will also help you unlearn those inner notions you believe, which create disharmony in you."

Through breath work, I could meditate deeply, become vulnerable in a safe space, and release much of the emotional stress of earlier pain and illness. In that safe space, I was the little girl Concha. Every deep breath took me deeper into the recesses of my mind. Painful episodes in my life surfaced. I recreated them mentally so that I could reach forgiveness in a loving environment.

Initially, the skeptical part of me dismissed the process because I didn't experience the miraculous remission of physical symptoms that I imagined would result.

"Don't be too attached to the external miracles," Luis reminded me. "Miracles happen at mind level."

"Do you mean that I have to see things differently?" I asked.

"How we think about ourselves and our circumstances is either conceived as separate or connected to our spirituality," responded Luis.

"Do you mean that when something bad happens to us, it may not be negative if we don't see it that way?"

"That's a simplistic way of saying it," he affirmed.

"Mom taught me the refrain that she always heard as a child: '*No hay mal por cual bien no venga*.' ('There's no bad thing from which something good won't come of it.')"

I was beginning to see what Luis meant by miracles. The biggest miracle was that I was beginning to believe Luis and the spiritual readings. A new belief requires us to shift how we perceive a situation—from a place of connection to our inner spirit rather than wishing for a big bang to happen out there. A number of events took place that convinced me that miracles were more than something in the mind.

Early one fall, two days after traveling to Los Angeles to collect research data, I was alone in the house. At about 4:00 a.m. on a Thursday, I was jolted awake by a sharp pain in my heart so intense that it impaired my breathing. Within seconds, the pain traveled swiftly, and I felt an explosion in the left side of my head. The pain throbbed near my heart, and a sensation of warm liquid seemed to drain from inside the left part of my head. It prickled like a hill of angry ants crawling down my face and arm. It itched deep inside my head, but I couldn't reach it to scratch. My entire left side was dead weight. Then I realized that I had a right arm and could use it to check. Trying to assure myself that I was too young for something like a stroke or heart attack, I tried to get up and find a mirror to see if my face was contorted, but I couldn't move. That's not supposed to happen until maybe forty years from now. Everything since the initial jolt seemed to have occurred at once. Maybe I'm dreaming, I thought. I glanced at the bedside digital clock with the large, bold numbers. It read 4:48 a.m. I didn't dare call and disturb loved ones. This was no nightmare. It seemed I was in the middle of a bizarre episode, foreign even for this body.

Lying still and counting one breath at a time, I waited, hoping that this stranger would pass. My years of meditation were being tested in a big way. I reached up to feel my face. It didn't feel crooked. However, a drooped face was the least of all the problems. By this point, shallow breathing made every breath painful, and my entire left side was immobile—paralyzed. It was now one hour into the episode.

Several minutes passed without any change. In dread, I wondered, should I call 911? Memories of the last time I had ended up in the emergency room made me hesitate to call my doctor. I remained in bed, hoping that I could make it till daylight and then call his office. I couldn't bear being jerked around by paramedics. Family and friends would insist that I call the hospital, but I had grown distrustful of hospitals. I didn't know what to do.

Then came the first positive thought: if I'm still thinking, I'm okay. Yet, something was wrong, no doubt of that. I reached for the phone, not knowing whom to call and dreading going to the hospital more than dying. But I remained calm. More than ever I saw the fruits of meditation, which were enabling me to observe and think before reacting. The neurologist came to mind. Stumbling to reach the phone with my right hand, pushing one button on the automatic dial pad, I called her.

"Help me, help me," I kept whispering into the phone. A male voice answered; sometimes other doctors were on call. I didn't care—I just wanted someone to talk with. I explained to him what I was experiencing. He quickly responded.

I whispered, "What can I do—can't breathe or move and something warm keeps dribbling down my face and arm. My whole left side is heavy and I can't move it."

"Dr. Sanders is at a conference out of town and I'm taking

her calls. She did leave your file here with me. Just a minute, let me read her notes." Then he continued, "From your history and what you're telling me, I suspect what you have is small blood clots, which may have originated in the heart area and were carried to the head, where they lodged. That happens with lupus," he continued. Given your history, I don't dare inject you with blood thinners because your system is likely to reverse the effects of the medication. If that happens, we have a big problem."

I listened and kept whispering, "Help me, help me" with an increasingly labored and debilitated voice. My mind vacillated between desperate fear and a detached peace, in which I was undisturbed by the events I was trying to control, quickly accepting that they were controlling me.

"Since I can't inject you with blood thinners, technically I can't put you in the hospital. The hospital isn't the best place for you anyway. I can't risk you getting weaker. I'm going to order a few tests that you can do on an outpatient basis so we can avoid admitting you to the hospital. I'll be ordering blood work, an EKG, an echocardiogram, an MRI, and a vascular sonogram to find out what's causing the problem."

"I'm scared," I whispered faintly.

"I know, and I'll try to get these tests pre-authorized with your insurance and scheduled right away so we can help you. Meanwhile, we're going to have to wait and hope that this doesn't worsen. Take two aspirins with a Zantac and try not to move too much."

"My left side is paralyzed. I'm scared," I repeated.

"I know, call me in one hour and report how you're doing."

He hung up. I was fading, unable to sit up in bed. I ran my fingers over the phone pad and dialed my sister Marie's number.

I thought she'd be awake since she usually left for the hospital at an early hour.

"What's the matter? I can barely hear you."

"Don't know. The neurologist thinks it might be debris carried to my head by small blood clots in the heart."

"Oh, my God. You were doing so well. What happened?"

"I'm scared."

"With good reason! I can't hear you. You better rest. Stop fighting, dear. We're all praying for you."

The neurologist on call was concerned enough to call about two hours later. He talked to the answering machine because I couldn't pick up the phone. He said, "I haven't heard from you, and I'm worried. If you're there, can you pick up the phone? When I've finished scheduling your tests, I'll call you again."

As soon as my right hand felt strong enough to push more than one button, I phoned Luis.

"What's going on?" he asked.

"I can't explain. Chest hurts," I gasped.

"You can do it, remember how to breathe from the diaphragm. Don't breathe from the chest. Breathe from the diaphragm."

Tears gushed from the depths of my soul.

"Good! Those are healing tears." Luis's words reassured me. "The one way out of your fear is through that tunnel."

"I'm fainting. Help me."

Luis's voice was barely audible in the background: "Know that you're safe, trust that you're being led to your place of healing."

His voice sounded distant, but it embraced me as if he were sitting next to me. He was right. I felt differently when I let go and trusted that I would be all right. I had to let go of trying to control this outcome. Maybe there was a reason why the doctor said he couldn't give me any medicine. Was I getting pushed to the edge to test my faith and lead me to my inner medicine? This was the ultimate test of what I had learned during the past four years: it's not what happens to us that's important; it's how we deal with it that makes the difference between suffering and remaining peaceful. We truly can't control many things in life, as I had once believed. I cried for what seemed like hours. Luis offered to take me to the doctor's office so I could take the tests.

"No. I'll be okay," I told him. I knew that I'd somehow find a way to get there. Suddenly I wasn't afraid at all. Nothing seemed to matter. I slept for a few minutes until the phone rang and awakened me. It was Dr. Sanders, the neurologist.

"How are you feeling?"

"My left arm and leg are still numb, but I can move them slightly, but the chest pain is still severe. I'm breathing a bit easier, but I'm still horribly debilitated."

"Okay, at least you're not worse. I arranged for your tests. You're to be at the hospital at eleven o'clock this morning."

"Fine."

Angels Around Me

How will I get there? I wondered. I can't worry. I don't have the energy. Whatever happens will be all right — somehow I knew that. At that moment the doorbell rang. It was Sandra, a dear friend. I had completely forgotten that she was coming over to work on our project. "You've got to take me to the hospital right now. I'm going for tests."

Sandra spent the entire day with me at the hospital. By the time she brought me home and helped me into bed, I couldn't think of calling anyone to organize transportation for the following day. Illness renders one unable to manage the details of self-care. When the body is unable, maybe that's when it's important to rely on our inner ability.

The following day, I faced the same dilemma of getting to the hospital to take the MRI — the one test that makes me nervous. As I'm somewhat claustrophobic, going into the tube with a steel mask half an inch from my face was more of a challenge than I could handle. I called my friend Nelva and could barely make myself heard, but she understood what I needed. She canceled her work at the office and took me to the exam. She held my hand and read me a favorite Alaskan story. Generous family and friends checked in throughout the day. I was extremely fortunate this way. Orchestration around the medical attention I needed felt effortless. Whether Eric was in or out of town, loved ones always stepped in to support me in every way.

When Dr. Barrett learned about my latest emergency, she called me.

"You were very, very lucky," she began. "No more steroids, or Methotextrate (the oral chemo medication). Suspend all medications and see me in three weeks. You've been through a lot."

"Yes, this has been very difficult."

"Rest and take care of yourself. Do you have someone who can help you?"

"Yes, I do."

Within days, I received the good news. The tests revealed no damage to my vascular system. I spent most of October in bed recovering. This was not how I imagined spending my quarter of sabbatical. Friends rotated taking me to appointments with the physical therapist and the acupuncturist. Someone was always showing up at my door with lovely flowers, a casserole, or a decadent dessert. On weekends, my sister Carmen arrived with armfuls of groceries, enough for an army. Without an appetite, I often forgot to eat. Nonetheless, I had faith that somehow all my needs would be met. The worst had passed and nothing mattered enough to worry. I couldn't even think straight enough to figure out what I needed from day to day. When people called to ask what I needed, nothing came to mind, so I told them to bring whatever they wanted.

One morning Berta called to ask if she could get me something from the store.

"I need toilet paper."

"Okay, I'll bring it to you tomorrow."

The next day Berta called again. "I can't bring the goods to you today because Raquel has the flu, and you don't need to be exposed to a virus. I'll come tomorrow to drop off the things. I won't come inside."

"Berta, don't worry."

On the day Berta was supposed to come, she called again. "You're not going to believe this, but my car is acting up and I can't make it across the Bay Bridge. I'm so sorry."

"I'm sure I have enough toilet paper around here — newspaper if necessary — no problem."

When the mail arrived later in the day, I looked outside the front door as I usually do. Oftentimes, the mailman left large packages on the doorstep. I opened the door and on the doorknob hung a sample roll of Charmin toilet paper. I brought the sample product in the house and laughed ecstatically. I thought, Okay, I get the message! I know you're taking care of me.

Getting back to work required major orchestration. One of the classes I taught was a joint doctorate seminar with students from California State University, Fresno. It required that I travel down to Fresno on alternate weekends. The students noticed how stressful this was for me. One Thursday, as I made the train reservations to get there, a student from one of my seminars called me. She said, "It seems that you're having a great deal of trouble commuting over here. My husband and I would like to pick you up in our private plane."

Initially I felt gut-wrenching fear about flying in a small plane, but then I heard myself say, "Of course. What airport will you use?"

"Buchanan Air Strip in Concord."

"Fine. What time?"

"He'll be there at three tomorrow afternoon."

"I'll get a ride there. Thanks so much."

The Cessna 100 arrived, and I became like an excited little kid on a pony for the first time. The spectacular views on this three-hour flight allowed me to see the world from a different place—much as I had been learning to do—and transcend from fear to clarity.

As miracles go, I've had many, and one of them I now live in. Facing the stress of failing health felt overwhelming enough, but added to that was increasing job stress and a disastrous financial crisis at home. The possibility of moving into a small studio was unappealing, yet I saw no other option. I began consulting the local papers, looking for a cheap studio in my neighborhood. Meanwhile, I fantasized about having a house in the hills with a lower mortgage payment—a fantasy quickly dampened by friends who learned of my secret wish. "Dream on," people told me. And then added, "You can barely make this house payment." I let myself feel disappointed, but quietly continued to search for a way out of financial disaster.

One Sunday afternoon I passed an OPEN HOUSE sign. Steering toward the curb to park and view the house, I was filled with questions. Why am I stopping here? I can't possibly buy a house until I sell mine, and I can't sell mine right now because the market is so bad. Ignoring the questions, I turned off the ignition and started toward the house. The several brick stairs leading to the front door made me question my motives. How could I possibly be interested in this place? I needed a one-level house with few if any stairs. After noticing that the house had an attached garage, I was encouraged to enter. It had a panoramic view of San Francisco, the Golden Gate Bridge, and other cities by the bay. Instantly I felt so comfortable that the owner and I sat in the living room and talked about everything except the sale price. When I was leaving, the owner handed me a price sheet. I was in disbelief at the incredibly low figure, and thought, I'll have to pay someone to take my house. Then, curiosity outweighed my pessimism.

I had nothing to lose by exploring every angle of financing. Jean, a friend in real estate, coached me through a wild escapade of finding a competent loan officer and accountant who were knowledgeable and creative, obtaining a win-win contract with the seller. Buying this home took on a life of its own. Every step tested my trust that if getting it were right for me, then everything I needed would be provided.

For two months, almost every day brought a new problem that left me wondering how I could handle it, but many of the developments had me believing that all the celestial bodies had aligned to facilitate this transaction. Overnight, something happened that I never could have predicted—interest rates dropped drastically. This qualified me for a very low fixed rate and a reasonable monthly payment. The timing was right for me as well as for the buyers who eventually bought my house in mid-winter, during a period when the real estate market was said to be "depressed" even in the Bay Area. Despite these conditions, the house still sold for a higher price than the home I bought. A total win-win deal unfolded all the way through the close of escrow.

I was nervous enough to hide this purchase from everyone until I had the key to my new home in hand. Then I invited friends to celebrate my birthday in my new, empty house overlooking the San Francisco skyline. Trusting the process with some detachment as to the outcome felt so liberating that I was challenged to live every day, practicing faith and gratitude.

Although I treasured my new home with its splendid views, there were moments when I missed the physical independence of past days. I looked forward to any small spurt of energy that enabled me to get out in the wheelchair. This made my family and friends nervous because of the steep hills around the neighborhood.

One sunny late-October afternoon, my thirst for a latte at my favorite neighborhood café overrode my common sense. I had grown impatient waiting for every kind heart in my world to help me attain normalcy. From my deck, I could see the four-block route I would take on Colusa Street. I put on jeans and a denim jacket, since it was cooling off. My friend Mary happened to call at the very minute I was grabbing the handrail to get myself out the door. She insisted, "Wait for me. I'll be there Saturday to help you. That's not something you want to do on your own."

I wanted my latte now, so I persisted and began my ride out of the garage, downhill one block, across Colusa, avoiding the steep slope on the hilly part of the street. Confident and in control of my Power-9000 chair, I continued on the sidewalk on Colusa, anticipating that first sip of a foamy latte. A lamppost in the middle of the sidewalk interrupted my smooth ride, forcing me into the street, which curved, keeping the afternoon traffic from seeing me. Thinking I could return to the sidewalk, I kept my hand on the gear, moving forward at 5 m.p.h. Then I noticed that the lampposts were set in the middle of the sidewalk every few yards. I had no choice but to forge forward in the street. Trembling with fear of ending up smeared on the pavement, I kept my eyes on the road and stayed close to the parked cars.

Half an hour later, I arrived, frazzled, at the café. Jim, noticing how shaken I looked, asked what had happened. After I related my story, he offered to drive me and the wheelchair home after he closed the café. I considered his offer as I sipped a latte and ate a bagel while reading the newspaper. After a shot of caffeine, the thought of waiting an hour for Jim became less attractive. I thanked him for the offer and then began the return trip on the opposite side of the street. I hugged the sides of parked cars, riding at a snail's pace until I approached that dreaded incline. Praying all the way, I pushed hard on the control. I made it to the very top, but then felt the wheels slipping. In my fantasy escape plan, if the chair failed me, I would throw myself onto the sidewalk and let the chair roll down without me. I made so many promises to God to get me up the hill that it'll take a lifetime to pay my debt, but I made it up and onto the sidewalk leading to my house! I vowed never again to risk an accident by trying to assert my independence. Just to make sure, I told friends about the incident so that they would remind me to exercise patience, and more important, faith. It was a miracle that I made it up the hill; I didn't need to repeat it.

Miracles are not things we wish for. They are inspired by our freedom from fear. When we let go of fear, we open up to being in the flow of life. I have experienced both—fear and the flow, as the people I needed appeared at exactly the right moment. Finding the Charmin sample hanging on my door-knob when Berta couldn't shop for me was a humorous confirmation of an integrated self. For me, that self confronted fear with the inner strength that Luis helped me tap while reaching out to the healers and friends to assist me with my body's needs. Being one with Spirit releases us from a sense of isolation and unites us with a community of love.

CHAPTER 7

Reading to the Soul

To think that our peace lives anywhere else
but within us is to relinquish our power.

My deepening faith built a stronger bridge between my spiritual community and me. After the episode that numbed my left side, a couple of friends insisted that I explore every available option for healing. They had attended a Pentecostal church, which held healing services. They invited me to attend a religious meeting in an Oakland church with a Pentecostal minister, Reverend Salazar. He was renowned for having healed many people, including some who were paralyzed in wheel-chairs; they got up and walked again. Initially, I was skeptical of attending a church that seemed so distant from my beliefs, but I respectfully accepted. "Nothing to lose," I said.

At the end of the two-hour Friday-night service, over a hun-dred people vacated the pews and waited in line to receive hands-on healing from the charismatic Rev. Salazar. And I was now ready for a big miracle! On this night I was the only one there walking with supports, and the eyes of the congregation followed me. I clutched my forearm crutches and waited my turn. The band played spirited rock music in the background as the reverend stood at the altar, placing his hands on people's heads, and stepping aside when they slipped into a graceful swoon. Their expression of faith reminded me of older Mexican women with gray *rebozos* draped around their heads, dragging themselves on their knees from the outside corners of the *catedrales* (cathedrals), making their way to the *Virgen de Guadalupe* icon. At the altar in each *catedral*, hundreds of testimonials to healing hung around the Virgin in the form of silver medallions signifying miracles granted.

Holding on to my crutches, I moved along with the line, getting closer to my turn to surrender. "Jesus, Jesus, you're my Lord!" came the wails of people with their gaze to the heavens, while others around them, accompanied by women assistants, lay whimpering on the dark-brown carpet at the altar. This I would later learn is called resting the spirit, something I felt my own life would not be complete without. For a moment, my trust turned to fear. I went as far as to imagine my neurologist being upset if I were to injure myself in search of Spirit. I turned to my friend who had brought me there. He smiled and clapped to the music.

Too late! It was my turn. The reverend came right up to me and placed his hands on both sides of my face. Leaning into my ear, he asked, "Do you accept the Lord into your life?"

"Yes," I said, but all I could think of was how much he needed mouthwash.

Looking down at my crutches, clearly disappointed that they had not dropped out from under me, he again prayed, "Let this be the beginning of your healing!"

"I've been praying for years, and I'm still ill," I told him, not wanting to let him off the hook so easily, but at the same time hoping he'd give me a magic potion to make the pain dissolve.

He moved his hands to the top of my head and prayed more: "Then let the healing continue from this point forward."

"Amen," I whispered.

Holding on to crutches, I walked out of the church the same way I walked in. To average eyes nothing had changed, but they could not have been more mistaken. No, I had not experienced spontaneous healing, but something much deeper had moved: I had a change of heart. In taking a chance, in risking, I had rediscovered the student within. My body had become my teacher and I was forced to pay attention. In the past, being a student had meant formulating and asking questions for the purpose of getting neatly wrapped answers and solutions. Now I inquired for the purpose of what the essayist Gloria Anzaldua calls living in the borderland, where ambiguity resides.

For me, that quest for learning is the oxygen that travels through my veins. Over the years, I've come to appreciate that learning is not about having to "know." The pursuit of knowledge is in the space of uncertainty. That's where we find the passion to keep going, keep searching, keep listening to that wise part of us that knows. I am challenged by the opportunity to see that there are no easy answers to important questions. In that unsafe borderland, I get to connect with others to create undreamed-of possibilities. Yes, physical health was still important to me as I left the Pentecostal church, but an internal shift was occurring. I wanted to heal my mind and spirit—to experience feeling quieter within. Getting physically well was no longer sufficient.

This was an important insight into who I really was and that I wanted to cure my soul. I no longer believed God was some umpire judging me from a seat on a mountaintop. I knew God was a Spirit residing in me. Knowing that I could tap into that Spirit within made me feel confident that healing was inevitable, and years later, I can affirm that this faith was fulfilled. If my body could heal through prayer, I wondered how it worked. How this would play out in days to come remained a mystery to me.

The church service filled my head with questions: What does prayer mean? Whom should I talk to? Am I talking to myself? Should I also be listening? Is listening part of prayer? Do we all want the same connectedness, forgiveness, and peace of mind? Is that what prayer offers us?

Answers to these questions resided in a niche that poetry touched within me. Like prayers, poetry tells the truth about the thing that matters most — our spirit. Valuing quiet contemplation gave me permission to take breaks from work and find a bit of solitude in my garden. I read poetry and books, gifts that friends had given me. Like prayer, poetry evokes feelings of peace and safety. Both embrace and shroud pain with words. Metaphors, allegories, and narratives paint pictures of pain as something challenging yet bearable. They turn us inward so that we will ever so gently touch our own pain. Poets write from the core of their being. They exalt and move the quality of life and humanity to center stage. Reading poetry became a personal prayer.

To feel more hopeful, I would have to rely on the familiar litany of prayers, the soft, kind words that were etched deep within, despite an afflicted body. The childhood notion of prayer as a magic wand that delivered results on demand gradually shifted. I began to understand how listening to the Divine had been the missing part of prayer. I prayed alone, with friends, in prayer groups, and in church, and when I couldn't attend Sunday service or evening meditations, my minister, Ken, visited me. Another peaceful space revolved around reading from spiritual works with Luis. The spiritual words became my sanctuary.

The impossibility of healing without a loving community became more apparent each day. Family and friends diligently shared their spiritual gifts with me, regardless of their religious beliefs. Everyone prayed for me. Inspirational messages wishing me good health arrived from Catholic, Jewish, Christian, Muslim, agnostic, and atheist friends. The depth of what this meant was not lost on me. What is it that we connect with when we wish healing for others and ourselves, regardless of our beliefs? Beyond religious affiliation, a bigger world transcends the body, where healing takes place. My loving community was intimately connected in that place. Phone calls, prayers, poems, and songs came from friends around the world: Spain, England, Mexico, Canada, France, and countless places in the US where I had lectured. The collective message was to trust. Sometimes I felt slightly embarrassed that so many people knew I was ill. Mostly, I felt blessed because I was learning to open myself up to receive the love others extended.

Close to home, I felt indebted to my family and friends, who frequently mobilized their church prayer groups on my behalf. My sister Lucy offered masses for my health at her neighborhood church. Other special moments came through phone calls. April, my goddaughter, only four years old at the time, called to tell me that she wanted to spend time alone with me the next time I came to Los Angeles.

I found solace in all that people did on my behalf, but at times impatience got the better of me. In these moments of emptiness and anxiety, I still doubted God and the benefits of prayer. Is healing His job? If God really cared, I would be well by now, I reasoned. Why doesn't this prayer stuff work for me? With little relief from what felt like an agonizing sentence, sometimes I distrusted the efficacy of any treatment.

Sometimes, when symptoms intensified and anguish overwhelmed me, I found refuge in the countless cards and letters from loved ones and friends that decorated the fireplace mantle. To counter these moments of total loss of control, I began a habit that anchored me to thinking differently. I lit a candle to remind myself that there was a God, somewhere, even if the evidence eluded me. Images of Mom lighting a quart-size candle in homage to her favorite saints when things got tough encouraged me. Mom's faith never waned. I had the benefit of this tradition of faith etched deep in me.

One Sunday morning, I looked forward to having brunch with a friend in San Francisco. Instead, feeling too debilitated to leave home, I canceled. In tears of desperation, I called my sister Marie in southern California. Her tears joined mine in frustration over my complications. Through gasping sobs and a winded voice I complained, "I can't breathe or move! I'm tired of medications and doctors and I want my life back. I don't know who I am anymore."

"We're on our way to church," Marie comforted me, "We'll ask our prayer group to pray for you."

That day the prayer circles multiplied with the phone calls I made to other friends, who in turn notified people they knew, and so on and so on. The prayer link spiraled across state lines. There is power in numbers. By early afternoon, I felt much stronger; I was able to sit up in bed and drink a cup of tea that a friend had prepared.

I had learned how to confront my darkness, transcend it, and experience joy. I had arrived at a point where I was consoled by the possibility that the distress of serious illness could not overcome me. Somewhere in me, a painless world existed. This belief alone made me feel stronger. I trusted that in that world I could outwit misery.

Healing Words

My private prayer sessions were sometimes mere tantrums, which progressively gave way to quieter conversations with my inner wisdom. I asked for understanding of what suffering meant in the context of my life. This required me to listen. Before this, the only listening I did was with my ears. From the first day of school, I learned that it was important to listen. Of course, it was the teacher's voice that carried the ultimate authority. Messages came through her words. "Turn to page thirty and do the problems before recess." There was no mistaking what was meant by such instructions.

My parents' voices also carried authority and naturally commanded a great deal of respect. I would never refuse to act on their directions: "Take the change from the wallet and go buy a half gallon of milk." The unmistakable sound of their voices reminded me that listening involved a different part of me—my heart. It meant lowering the volume of judgment in an effort to hear. It is in that quiet place, where a light flickered like a soft candle flame, that I heard a favorite healing word—faith.

I felt increasingly comfortable with language that focused me inward, and Luis's words were the strongest. I found myself less and less an outsider. "After all," Luis reminded me, "the immune system involves far more than its physical organs and tissues." I was familiar with Larry Dossey, Andrew Weil, and Bernie Siegel, medical doctors who spoke about the idea that our emotional, mental, and spiritual dimensions intertwine to support immune-system function.

Like prayers and poetry, music also spoke to the inner healer in me. A stressful workplace at the university made my home a haven more than ever. Although I still demanded more of my body than was realistic, I cherished the minutes of relaxation I made myself take. Listening to music caressed me like a loved one's tender hug. Momentarily, I sank into rhythms that cushioned the pain. Ballads, tangos, and *Mariachi* liberated me from my body. Audiotapes of popular *Mariachi* music arrived from my sister Lupe. They were enjoyable companions in the car. Imagining myself holding a cold beer on a balmy evening at the Plaza Garibaldi in Mexico City, listening to the guitars of *El Mariachi Sol de Mexico*, boosted my energy for several minutes. Quite different from *Mariachi*, Beethoven's *Ode to Joy* made me feel calm, as did Stevan Pasero's classical guitar.

Whenever I could get out to a favorite jazz place, I did. An evening of live music, a favorite form of recreation, was like getting a two-week vacation. When I wanted to sing along, women vocalists touched the feminine power in me. A friend recorded a tape for me with some of my favorite vocals, including *Gracias a la Vida*, Barbra Streisand's *Memory*, Bette Midler's *Wind Beneath My Wings*, and Sara Vaughn's *Prelude to a Kiss*. For a precious few minutes, song could penetrate deeper than the stabbing, burning joint and muscle pain. My musical interlude ended with the audiotape, and my consciousness returned to the body—now my familiar home.

This painful body, too, needed to be expressed. In the kitchen,

I could no longer hold the dishes. Tears, tears, and more tears followed the plates and glasses that dropped from my hands onto the floor. Now I had double the work—sweeping up a mess of broken dishes. Getting a broom, moving it from side to side, and bending down to hold the dustpan to collect the shards took almost an hour on this particular day. Just then, Eric walked into the kitchen with a bag full of groceries. Without a word, he took the broom and finished cleaning up.

My feelings of resentment were less about the broken glass and more about the hours of reading and grading a stack of student papers that awaited me. Through tears, I shouted curses against God for abandoning me! Eric held me until I stopped sobbing. Dinner out after that catharsis was a welcome remedy to a frustrating ordeal.

These distressing episodes reminded me that healing meant more than good feelings. A crucial part of healing was to be able to express those feelings that I usually categorized as "bad."

Comfort also came from daily calls from loved ones. Talking to my nieces and nephews in Los Angeles was the best medicine of all. They reminded me to connect with the joy around me. Hearing their voices, I could put things in perspective. Mickey and Marco, niece and nephew, called regularly. Their stories usually provided a bit of humor. One evening, the phone rang.

"Concha," came the familiar child's voice, "I got a certificate for best speller in my class today." It was Mickey, my niece, seven years old at the time.

"That's great, Mick, what did you spell?"

"I spelled 'enormous' and 'meticulous.' The other kids couldn't spell them."

"Congratulations, dear! What do those two words mean?"

"We don't have to know that yet. Bye, Concha."

Luis, too, called often. His support never failed me. He encouraged me to think about the meaning of my illness. "Using the body for purposes other than the extension of love creates disease," he explained.

I did not like the sound of that! Was he saying that I had not been a loving person and that was why I became ill? I certainly didn't need to be blamed for not loving. I knew better; I felt closer to loved ones and to building active, literate communities than ever before.

I told Luis that my life had been meaningful. I merely wanted the pain and debilitation to cease! "That's not much to want, Luis."

He laughed gently and added, "Understand, Concha, I am not saying you haven't loved. I mean that illness can be our guide for deeper love and peace."

"How could disease ever bring me love or peace?" I scoffed. Luis answered firmly but compassionately, challenging a long-held belief that the body was merely a machine at my command. I sincerely wanted to understand Luis.

Frequent calls from friends were a welcome safety net. I always looked forward to hearing from Berta whose calls had become a welcome ritual. Laughing released endorphins and helped me ignore the pain.

Regardless of the illness, a celebration is great medicine. On a Saturday afternoon one July, three strolling guitarists strummed bolero tunes for me while over a hundred loving friends and family members enjoyed the festivities as we celebrated my promotion to full professor. Three and a half years into a health condition that had choreographed more rhythms than a ballroom dance, I stood at the threshold of another turning point.

On crutches, I rambled from table to table, indulging in the laughter and hugs from everyone.

Laughter, music, and loved ones were special medicine. A pained body held the memories of the day as I drifted off to sleep. In dreams I saw myself, in a long, flowing gown, dancing gracefully down the same bike path where I once walked routinely for an hour every morning. I awakened encouraged with the thought that one day I would again dance without a cane! Before this, I had expected to get well so I could continue working. Now I wanted to get well for no reason other than to experience a symptom-free body. Whether in pain or not, I sought a peaceful mind.

CHAPTER 8

Appreciating Healers

Our body is precious.
It is a vehicle for awakening.
Treat it with care.

— Buddha

Each step toward healing took as much conscientious effort as learning English when I first immigrated to California and entered the second grade. Whether it was consulting a *curandera* (traditional Mexican folk healer), a Chinese acupuncturist, or Dr. Barrett, I was aware of how lifelong beliefs about the body and illness do not change overnight. After all, I had spent many years believing that the body was designed to work on my command. Caring for our health requires reading, studying, and researching new ideas and practices that can help us understand our condition. Without sufficient time to rest, medical complications escalated rapidly, requiring countless hours in doctors' offices. In their waiting rooms, I spent hours designing a health plan with multiple healing modalities.

Although I continued to work with Dr. Barrett, I remained open to every healing tradition that could help me get stronger.

Dr. Barrett suggested changing the type of chemo I was taking in hopes of getting my immune system to respond. Would going from Lukeran (an oral medication) to Methotextrate (a different kind of oral medication) strengthen me? Would I betray my last decision not to accept steroid treatment in addition to chemo? It's possible to damage one's health while trying to heal it. But Luis's sensible words kept me steady. "You can or cannot take the drugs. That's not important. What matters is how you think about yourself regardless of your decision."

"You mean I can choose the drugs without violating my previous decision not to take more drugs?"

"Whatever you do, stay focused on your oneness with Spirit. You're already whole, and no drug can make you less or more whole. You're not judged as weak if you do, nor are you less loved, either way."

Day after day, the steroids and chemo drugs swirling in my body conspired to keep me awake most of the night. After only two hours of sleep, I lay in bed with one thing to do: talk to God.

Hello, I'm here again. I'm grateful for another day that I can talk to you. I know I complain a lot because my body isn't working right now. I have faith that you're helping me to recover completely, minute by minute. Maybe right now isn't the time to ask what you want me to do once I'm fully recovered, but sometimes I can't help but wonder what gifts you have in store for me. Selfish, I know. Maybe I should be grateful for the love that surrounds me. Still, I wonder, is there something more I should be doing?

Long hours of silence followed my monologues.

Luis did not judge me when I told him that I continued to pursue instant miracle cures. However, he always reinforced the idea that I had to be my own health guru down an uncharted path where no rules existed. This meant acknowledging and trusting that whisper within.

Relying on unconventional healing practices reminded me of ancestral ways. Long before modern medicine, before the wizardry of high-priced drugs, people in ancient cultures sought solutions for illness through natural means. As a young girl, I learned about Mexican *sobadores* (bone healers) whom my parents sought for sprains and strains. *Sobadores*, who learn their healing arts by apprenticing with elders, reset bones using herbal oils. In college, friends and I went to a *curandera*. I knew well the practice of *curanderismo*, Mexican herbal healing and the use of a broom to cleanse one of illness or other suffering, so I felt comfortable visiting Señora Romero, a *curandera* recommended by my friend Amalia.

Señora Romero was in her sixties, with salt-and-pepper hair tied in one thick braid around the top of her head. Tall and short herb bushes hugged her one-bedroom, white stucco house. She greeted me at the door and asked me to enter and wait in the tiny living room area adorned with an elaborate altar. Short, flickering candles shone beneath the carvings and pictures of three saints. This familiar scene I knew well from the many candles I had lit in Catholic churches. Mom had told me that the Catholic Church frowned on *curanderismo* practices. I wondered why that was the case, since this was a sanctuary much like many churches where I had prayed.

While I waited for Señora Romero, I realized that I actually knew little about this particular *curandera*'s ritual. One thing was for certain, I wanted a miracle — to be free from the illness that was wrecking my life. Maybe this time I would drop my cane and leave her house with the upright, strong, and pain-free body I remembered.

Curtains parted as she entered from her back room after about fifteen minutes. She told me that she had been pray-ing for me before my arrival and that her saints had advised her to accept me for a healing because I needed help. She cer-tainly had that right. Vulnerable in her presence, my eyes felt warm with tears, and I began to cry. She sat close to me, took my hand, and held it until I regained my composure. In a faint voice I asked, "What do the saints say is the problem?"

"Don't be afraid," she said, "You'll be fine." She asked me if I believed in God. I said yes. Then she motioned for me to fol-low her into the back room. Walking behind her, I had mixed feelings about being there. On the one hand, I felt totally trust-ing of whatever this mysterious ritual might hold. On the other hand, I felt skeptical and critical. If I was going to benefit from this visit, I had to make an agreement with myself to keep an open mind.

Walking into Señora Romero's back room was like becoming part of her altar in the living room. Everywhere I turned, a dif-ferent saint stared back. She motioned me to sit in a large, com-fortable-looking navy-blue seat while she lit the incense. The scent brought back memories of the seven-year-old Concha in a Catholic Church, waiting in line for communion and feeling woozy from the all-consuming smoke. Señora Romero began a litany of prayers as she approached me with what looked like the bottom of a broom. She waved a smoking herbal stick up and down around me, reciting prayers in Spanish. One that I heard louder than others said, "*El espiritu de Dios te cuida y cura. Nada te vencera."* ("Spirit is taking care of you. Nothing can hurt you.") Her healing words conveyed trust that all was well. I felt safe.

A few times, she lapsed into speaking tongues, which I recognized from the Pentecostal churches I had visited. I wondered what I should do, then closed my eyes and visualized myself perfectly healthy in mind, body, and soul! For the short time that she prayed over me, I felt peaceful. It was like being in a deep meditation, interrupted only by the dense incense smoke that filled the room.

When she finished praying, she motioned me to return to the living room and wait. After a couple of minutes, she came out holding a package of rose-scented herbs. She instructed me to prepare a bath nightly for a week and soak in the herbs. She then motioned me to drop a donation in the plate labeled DONATIONS. As I walked to the door, I heard her say, *"Siga con su fe y amor."* ("Move forward from a place of faith and love.") With cane in hand, I left Señora Romero's house feeling relaxed and a bit more peaceful than when I arrived.

Although I still used a cane to help me walk out of Señora Romero's home, I knew that her ritual had been healing. Her prayers returned me to familiar childhood days of sacred words conveying strong faith. Her words telling me to trust that nothing could hurt me encouraged me along my healing track.

With profound faith and hope, I continued pursuing a variety of non-Western healing traditions, especially Chinese medicine. I was no stranger to Chinese medicine, so I felt comfortable with it. Years before, I had experimented with it for other medical concerns. I also felt a special connection to the tradition because my maternal grandfather was of Chinese background. However, I had never openly acknowledged this part of my

ancestry. I returned to my Chinese roots for a chance at wellness. This silent part of my Chinese heritage found a voice in
my healing through my appreciation of Chinese culture and
healing practices.

The roots of Chinese medicine run deep; the practices of
acupuncture and specialized herbs are based on 4,000 years
of knowledge and history. I couldn't argue with that. Although
I had done acupuncture before, I didn't know the medicinal
principles on which herbal and acupuncture treatments were
based. Again, as in the early years of learning a new language, I
tried to understand what Chinese medicine meant. This time,
the teacher listened to my story and patiently showed me how
to read *Between Heaven and Earth*, a book on Chinese medicine, one page at a time. Another promise of Chinese herbs
is their nurturing properties, which strengthened my energy
rather than depriving me of it.

I felt at home straddling conventional Western and Eastern
medical-care philosophies. I dreaded most doctors' appointments, yet appreciated my doctors' interest in me. But I most
looked forward to acupuncture sessions with Dr. Green. After
four treatments within one month, my energy level and physical movement improved. For me, acupuncture healed when
the chi—the life force that runs through us—moved.

Feeling somewhat more stable, I began doing tai chi daily.
It became my new dance, integrating body and mind. Performing the slow, graceful 166 movements required enormous
strength. Five minutes at a time was all I could do. Still, one
gentle stretch at a time, my stamina increased, and after several months of class I was standing and doing tai chi for half
an hour. My experience, as well as research, convinced me of
the merits of tai chi.

A research study reported on a group of 4,000 senior citizens who were observed over a few years. The group who did tai chi had significantly fewer falls and hip fractures than the group that didn't. Tai chi helps strengthen the neurological system, as well as the muscular, skeletal, respiratory, and circulatory systems. I felt stronger and more energetic, and had a steadier sense of balance. Tai chi echoed the lessons explicit in quantum physics and in philosophical and spiritual readings: that we exist in a relational plane where there is no objective world that separates us from each other. The healing language of tai chi was not in words, but in the powerful, strengthening motions and the freedom I felt while moving.

Neither Western, Mexican, nor Chinese medicine offered permanent solutions for the rapacious, unpredictable illness camped in my body. More than ever, I wanted to understand how mind, body, and spirit intersected to heal the body.

Adding to the package of complementary healing practices, I began Reiki meditation with two teachers, Camilo and Olga, who were masters in Reiki energy work. Reiki was a simple practice to accept. It didn't require me to believe anything different. Reiki shares similarities with Chinese medicine in that it works with the body's flow of energy through gentle, hands-on touch. The basic tenets of Reiki have roots in the Japanese Buddhist tradition, which was already a part of my spiritual repertoire. "Rei" means wisdom or higher power, and "ki" is life force.

Reiki treatments combine both of these energies, creating a feeling of relaxation, security, and peace. Each time I had a treatment I felt a calming radiance flowing through me. Daily Reiki practice helped subdue the pain, allowing me to regain some of my energy. It helped me feel more connected to myself and others. I benefited physically, emotionally, and spiritually. A major tenet of Reiki involves the person taking an active part in their healing. I learned the language of responsibility for my own healing. I committed to healing through whatever modality I responded to.

From *curandera* to Reiki, the various healing practices shared an important principle: They all emphasized living in harmony with our surroundings by integrating mind, body, and spirit. Depressurizing our lives in this complex world sometimes feels like more pressure. Feeling in control of our personal and professional environment is critical for a low-stress life. In our culture, however, keeping a full calendar has come to be identified with "being important." Our workaholic tendencies keep us stuck in a frenzied pace. Although I maintained a busy schedule even while in a power wheelchair, my perception of disability changed: I was no longer a "disabled body" unable to move quickly. Rather, I was a person moving at a gentler pace.

Pacing my daily and weekly activities balanced and energized me. I could read a student's dissertation in two hours, a task that previously consumed eight. This meant more time to play. Professional women who have made breakthroughs in male-oriented workplaces have taught each other conscious and assertive behavior. Setting limits, however, had not been part of my emancipation. Pacing now became a critical component. I reconnected with those ideals that nurtured me while composing new thoughts and discovering new words like joy.

My new language enabled me to set reasonable limits on work. Reluctant to say no, I had been trapped in a ferocious routine of hard work and hard play. While at the time that seemed normal, I now felt the toll it took on my health. Intellectually

and physically, I knew that I could no longer perform like the
lightning rod I had been. I had overextended myself countless
times, changing physical therapy appointments, going without
breakfast, lunch, even water, just to get to a scheduled university meeting on time. I would arrive at the designated place on
time only to find that the folks who had insisted that I meet
with them arrived nearly a half-hour late. They were still having lunch. This made me furious. Often I wished that I had
the carefree sensibility about time that many people stereo-
typed Mexicans as having—"Mexican time." Going with the
flow seemed the graceful, stress-free way to go.

So I made some changes. For as long as I could recall, I had
accommodated people's requests for meeting times at the office.
Making health a top priority, my new language sounded more
like this: "I can't meet with you; I have a conflict on that date."
I thought of many guiltless ways to say, "No, I can't right now."
Before committing to more meetings, I rehearsed the state-
ments that had always been used on me.

"I'll think about it."

"I'm sorry, I have to postpone our meeting."

"I'm sorry, I'll have to cancel our appointment."

"I'll be late for the session."

"I'll get back to you."

"I have a conflict on that day."

This reframing gave me a chance to schedule the days so that
I didn't crowd myself just to please others. The more I drew
those boundaries between unnecessary work and myself, the
easier it became.

At my home office, I wrote reports, made calls, faxed letters,
held phone conferences, and e-mailed many people across the
country. Even the dining room was part of my office space, as

I had conferences with students who came to discuss their research. Trips to the university were reserved for teaching, keeping office hours, and faculty meetings. Setting limits modified my lifestyle. This was a form of "Mexican time" that worked for me.

Relearning to Walk

In early autumn, I found myself having to recall the *curandera*'s words, "Move forward from a place of faith and love," as I had a totally unforeseen setback. Fall breezes blew in a new school year as predictably as the leaves changed color, but I found myself in a different kind of classroom this autumn.

After a morning shower, I began working. I fixed a second cup of coffee and began tackling a new laptop PowerBook that had frustrated me for days. Sitting, holding the laptop, a sudden weakness overcame me. I felt like I was fainting. My heart raced out of control and I went limp. Breathing slowly, I managed to compose myself and resumed writing. An hour later, my heart again throbbed uncontrollably. I tried walking to the desk, but bumped into the door frame as I grabbed the phone from the desk to call the paramedics. Within minutes, they arrived, immediately strapping an oxygen mask on my face.

A short ride later, I was in the emergency room. From the gurney, I had one view, the dull blue curtain that closed around my cubicle, separating me from the bed next to mine. I could hear a woman's soft voice over the loudspeakers, paging doctors. The hands of the nurse standing next to me moved quickly, stretching out my arm to insert a needle for the IV drip hanging on a pole. The cold, sticky, round patches that they plastered on my chest were familiar. An EKG was in progress. "Your heart looks fine," came the nurse's voice, which by now sounded as faint as my breath.

"Your family doctor called and told us that you have a history of lupus."

"Yes," I gasped, as the emergency-room doctor entered.

"Has this happened before?"

"Yes," I gasped again.

"Hang in there. We'll figure out where the problem is," the doctor said. "I suspect you might be having a relapse."

I closed my eyes, fantasizing that any minute the doctor would come back and tell me that they had a new pill to eliminate all of my body's ailments. I clung to memories of innocent times when music and dance were the day's preoccupation. Little did I know that this trip to the emergency room would turn into the longest hospital stay since I became ill.

Hours after my arrival at the ER, the wait continued. "God!" I pleaded with shallow breath, "I've been strong without medications for two years. This can't be a relapse!" The loudspeaker blared, asking a doctor to report to the emergency room. This was no small faint that had landed me in the hospital. I knew I was in deep trouble. I was smack in the middle of a full-blown relapse and this could be the final curtain. "I'm scared. You've seen me through many tough times with this illness. I'm here again. Wasn't it supposed to get better if I had faith? Maybe I don't know how this faith thing works, but I don't have anything else to cling to right now. I'm giving it all up to you. Help me!" Eyes closed, I whispered to myself, wishing to feel Mom's comforting hand that was always there in tough times. "God, if you get me through it, I am yours. I promise to trust you. You will hear from me, not only in hard times but every single day. I want you to guide me always. I don't know what more to do."

With no answers about my condition, I stared at the pale-blue curtain. Supplications to God came from a place much more hopeful than my weak vocal cords could utter. With barely enough muscle strength to clutch my forearm crutches, I didn't know where such faith would come from. But a younger Concha knew. The sweet, chubby, eight-year-old girl with austere brown eyes and short, wavy, black hair was determined to get through this crisis. That little girl whose faith had seen her through tough times would once again guide me to find the trust I needed.

Desperate for a solution I clung to every clue around me. One thing is certain: there's little privacy in hospitals. Voices came through the thin curtains drawn between the emergency-room beds.

"Where are your veins?" came the nurse's voice.

"Gone. I shoot up drugs," answered the woman on the bed next to mine.

"How can we draw blood?"

"Use the bottom of my left foot."

A male doctor's voice entered my space and jarred me back into my own drama. "What seems to be the problem?" asked the doctor who walked in and sat in a chair across the room.

"Weak, in pain," I whispered.

"I can't hear you. Speak up, please."

"I can't."

"I'll be back in a minute. You rest," he said. And walked out. There I was, alone with my thoughts.

What felt like an eternity later, the doctor returned. "Your chart says that you have a history of lupus. Correct?"

"Yes."

"Do you think you might be having a relapse?"

"I don't know," I responded.

He continued his probing. "Your potassium is quite low, so we're starting an IV and may need to have you take the potassium orally as well. What's this that the nurse says about you thinking you might be allergic to hair color?"

"I'm not sure," I said. "Maybe I fainted because I used hair color."

"You think you fainted because of the hair color?"

Barely able to whisper, I pointed to my hair and tried to tell him that I had used hair coloring that morning.

Sitting at the corner of the room quite a distance from me, he called out, "What? Speak up! I can't hear you. Why are you pointing to your hair?" Finally, he got up and came to the bedside. He leaned down to hear me and I pointed to my hair and I said, "Hair color."

"What? Oh, your hair. Yes, yes, it looks nice," he said, obviously thinking I was fishing for a compliment.

Again I whispered, "No, no. Maybe I fainted because of the hair color."

"Is this a new chemical product you used?" the doctor asked.

"No. It's a natural herbal tint." Although I heard myself say that it was natural, I distrusted anything at this point that might be the culprit of this flare-up.

"You don't have a rash, which usually signals an allergic reaction," he reassured me.

"Okay," I whispered, wondering, then what?

The doctor continued, "The hair color didn't cause the faint or weakness and pain. You're probably having a lupus relapse."

The confusion about whether or not the hair color had caused the SLE relapse got me thinking about how it all began.

Planning to attend a friend's wedding in a few days, earlier that day I tinted my hair. When the paramedics arrived, I mentioned to them that I had used the hair color, thinking that maybe the chemicals in the tint had caused me to feel faint. They, in turn, relayed that information both to my doctor and to the emergency-room staff. There developed a series of humorous events related to the state of my condition and its possible connection to the hair color. In any other setting, I wouldn't have given this levity any attention, but in this case it became a lighthearted distraction from the serious matter I knew was unfolding.

When I arrived at the emergency room, the paramedic had announced me by name to the person I knew as a voice behind the desk. The woman responded, "Oh, yes, the hair-color lady." A few minutes later, I recognized the same voice as that of the ER nurse inserting the IV.

Taking my medical history, the nurse continued, "How old are you?" I told her my age, and from the corner of my eye, I could see her do a double take.

"You certainly wear it well."

I motioned to her to get closer and then I whispered, "It's the hair color." She didn't laugh, but suggested, "Maybe next time you'll have it done professionally."

In the emergency room, waiting for the potassium, I began to think about work, wondering when I could return to the university. But even the word "work" was elusive. What would work mean after this?

From the emergency room, the nurses moved me to the acute-care unit. They continued administering heavy dosages of potassium intravenously and orally in liquid form in a paper cup to stabilize my heart palpitations. Although the potassium kept me from fainting again, I felt like I had been injected with kryptonite. There were so many times in my past when I'd wished I could just lie still and have someone take care of me. Now I was still, and medical attendants were caring for me. Be careful what you wish for. That night they admitted me into the hospital.

The following day, Dr. Barrett came into the room and stood next to the bed. "Your heart stabilized with the potassium."

"I eat a banana every day. Why do I need to get more potassium in an IV and orally?'

"You'd have to eat several bushels to make up for the amount you lost. Now we need to get you on steroids and chemo along with intense physical therapy to reduce inflammation and strengthen your muscles."

"No! No drugs, I can't handle them," I objected.

"You have the right to refuse medication, but you need to know that I wouldn't do this unless I was pressed to. Right now your muscles are not responding, and we've got to work aggressively to jump-start your system with everything we have."

I turned into the pillow, hiding the tears from her. I felt like I was in a flashback of five years earlier, when I was first diagnosed with lupus; medical specialists bombarded me with heavy meds, which frightened me. I thought of Luis's words—that in healing we do not go back to where we were before. Flare-ups feel like setbacks, but we can use them as opportunities to grow and discover other parts of our life. Now, this new occasion was about getting through all the therapies for as long as it took to make me self-reliant again so that I could care for myself at home. I was grateful for one thing: my prayers had been answered. The decision to take drugs had been made. I had taken one step around the corner.

"Don't get upset," came Dr. Barrett's firm voice. "You need all your strength and sprit to help us stay on track."

Her words comforted me like the smell of my mother's fresh, hot flour tortillas throughout the house on rainy days. Unable to do anything else, I fixed my eyes on the sanitized white ceiling, lying quietly like so many times before when words seemed futile.

If it was rest I needed, the hospital was not the place where I would get it. When the lights went out, the cold darkness in my room magnified the sounds and noise in the hallway: elevators beeping, phones ringing, dishes clanging, water running, shoes squeaking, carts rolling, women talking and laughing, even people's clothes swishing when they walked near my door, which remained open all night. Just when I thought silence had arrived, the loudspeaker blared, "Maggie Morris, please pick up line three. Maggie Morris, line three, please."

"Lights out. It's 10:00 p.m.," ordered the nurse.

"I'm hungry. My stomach is growling."

"Would you like a little apple juice?"

"Can you get me something, fruit or bread?"

"Sorry, the kitchen is closed. The juice offer still holds."

"Juice it is."

Why does the dark magnify pain? How was it possible that the third-degree burn pain enveloping my body felt even more intense now? Sleep did not come when the lights went off. I wanted to turn on the radio or the TV to screen out the reminders that I lay in a strange bed. How could I stop worrying about what would happen to me tomorrow? How long would I have to take chemo and steroids? I wanted to be able to work again, but right now I was too weak to function normally, much less work as fiercely as before. Now Spirit would have to work for my body.

Following a one-night stay on the acute treatment floor, the nurses transferred me to a private room in a skilled-care building for intense physical therapy. Spirit was already hard at work. The private room was the only one available, and for once, my insurance was willing to pay for something that accommodated me.

From the hospital bed in my new private room, I had a fabulous view of the East Bay hills. Nurses, therapists, and housekeepers came and went, helping to make me comfortable. I rested, watching the foot traffic carrying water pitchers, trays, towels, and one flower arrangement after another.

A week into the hospital stay, I felt like a new kid, able to take my first steps.

"It's wonderful to see that you're in good spirits in spite of the difficult situation," said Ken, who came to pray with me one morning.

"It's not hard with so many loving calls and visits. It tires me sometimes, but I think it's the best medicine I can get. Here comes the tough part of the therapy."

Debra, the physical therapist, had entered the room.

"Hello, Debra, this is Ken."

"Concha, we're going for a walk today."

"I won't argue with you."

"Can I stay to watch?" Ken asked.

"Yes, I can use a cheerleader," I said.

"From the bed, let's make the doorway your destination. I'm holding on to your belt, so you won't fall."

My feet dragged. I shuffled two steps. "That's all," I told her.

"You're dragging your feet. That doesn't qualify as taking steps."

"What's a step?"

"Lift the front of your right foot." I raised my entire leg. "No, that's your leg. Lift the front of your foot up."

"I can't feel my feet from the ankles down, so I don't know what they're doing."

"Let's strap these elastic leg braces on you. They connect your feet to your legs. They're giant rubber bands. You pull on them as I hold you."

"Oh, you mean like a marionette?"

"When I instruct you, you pull them up and down."

Lift, forward, heel, front, down. Lift, forward, heel, front, down. Lift, forward, heel, front, down—the therapy continued for an hour. In the night's quiet, I rehearsed Debra's instructions—lift, forward, heel, front, down. Maybe memorizing the words would help me remember. It's like mapping the steps to a new dance, I thought. When I'm rehearsing a belly dance or learning a new salsa step, I map it out mentally before practicing it on the floor.

Tears of exhaustion dribbled from the corners of my eyes onto the pillow, but I was feeling more confident. I had managed before and I could do it again. I trusted in the body's resilience.

Alone at night at the end of this peaceful Sunday, my eyes were fixed on the window. The dim streetlights dotted the East Bay hills. My body continued to hold the attention of all the medical attendants because of what it could not do. I felt grateful, however, for every new step I took. I had faith in more than the physical therapy I received.

Through personal visits, phone calls, cheerful cards, and carts filed with flowers, support poured in from loved ones across the country, tempering the impatience that sometimes still got the better of me. Every person's flowers and cards expressed the love I counted on. Bouquets of gladiola, daisies, and pink stargazing lilies filled the room with their sweet scent. With my muscles immobile, my inner strength worked overtime. Staring out the window, I was filled with love for the Bay Area, my home.

Another special treat arrived five out of seven days of the week: it was Maria, the housekeeper, whom I affectionately nicknamed "the broom lady." She reminded me of a *curandera* using a broom to dispel all illness and distress from a person. Maria did more than clean rooms. She entertained me with her stories in Spanish. "I don't know why I find it so easy to talk to you, since I don't even know you. Usually, I just sweep and keep quiet. But you seem very nice."

"Thank you. I enjoy your stories," I said.

"It's what I've lived." Pushing her big black broom, she continued talking. "My parents owned a tortilleria in Zacatecas, Mexico. It was there that Mother taught me how to work. She taught me that the tortilla was life's substance. You see, the tortilla is made of earth's best—the corn, so how could we go wrong making the tortilla part of our meals?"

Maria sure had it right: coming from the people of the corn meant that we were of strong stock. With her stories, this woman with a broom brought my grandmother and mother to mind. Grandma was from Zacatecas, and Mom's name was Maria. Their healing spirit was present when Maria cleaned my room, her stories transforming her broom into a *curandera*'s. I felt the strength of her healing presence.

When I was only a few days away from returning home after the long hospital stay, the physical and occupational therapists increased our sessions. They worked tirelessly at teaching me to do what I had once taken for granted. Julie, the occupational therapist, helped me strengthen my wrists and fingers so I could hold my fork. She came into my room daily after the physical therapist had finished with her routine. The occupational therapy workout began with three plastic containers filled with hard putty, which I was to hold, squeeze, and shape into long rolls resembling taquitos. I fantasized about being able to use my laptop and write with a pen.

Every morning began the same way: after breakfast, Julie pushed me up to the occupational therapy room on the sixth floor in a wheelchair for occupational therapy. "Let's see you get up from the chair and carefully walk on your crutches to the sink," she instructed me. "Now pour water into the plastic container, walk back here to the microwave, and boil the water."

"Okay," I responded. Waiting three minutes for the water to boil, I held on to my crutches, looking out the window that faced San Francisco. For a moment, I felt desperately homesick and excited all at once. I missed relaxing on the back deck, gazing out to the bay. Suddenly, remembering how strong I'd grown since entering the hospital put a smile on my face.

New Healing Directions

Home. It had never felt so sweet to sleep in my own bed. Staring out at the spectacular San Francisco skyline from my bedroom window, I treasured the amazing view. I was not only comfortable in the familiar physical surroundings, but I also felt peaceful in that place within, which I had grown to trust like a sanctuary.

To assist the healing progress, I took an administrative leave from the university. I heard the clock ticking especially loud because the university agreed to the leave with the stipulation that I would return to full-time professorship at the end of six months. I had to believe it was possible.

Stretching, pulling, and reaching to build stamina consumed long hours of each day. I took oxygen for two hours a day to help my diaphragm and chest muscles breathe when they were too debilitated to do their job. On alternate days, the physical therapist came to the house. She stretched me beyond the comfort point with rigorous exercises. It was a good kind of pain, like what you feel at the end of a marathon — you're pained and exhausted but you've crossed the finish line. Her visits continued for several months, then tapered off until she felt that I could use the wheelchair to go to the medical center for treatments.

My needs around the house were taken care of by loved ones, especially my sister Carmen. She had neatly arranged all the groceries in the cupboards so that I could reach them. I accepted my friend Beatriz's offers to do the laundry and clean the house. To create wheelchair access between the bedroom and kitchen, a contractor tore down a wall and installed French doors. Wheeling myself into the kitchen to make coffee without a major obstacle became reason enough to wake up every morning.

From sunrise to sunset, scheduled meditation, prayer, and plenty of bed rest consumed me. Major changes unfolded: walls came down between rooms inside my house while fences went up in my relationship with Eric. For me, healing meant redefining my relationship to spirituality, body, loved ones, and work. The time had come to reconsider my relationship with men in general. I was undergoing purposeful changes, and I expected Eric to come along. However, we do not always get our heart's desire.

Eric and I had been moving in different directions for a long time, but the drama of my illness kept us from making firm decisions about our respective careers. Now it was time for both of us to let go. Although our decision was mutual, I blamed myself for the separation. Would we have been able to work things out if I was not ill? I crashed under the anger, fear, anxiety, and loss until I heard a tender voice say, "You're okay."

It would take some time after our separation for us to let go, forgive, and again become friends. Interestingly, pain—whether in the joints, muscles, or emotions, can transform us at the deepest levels if we turn it over to Spirit. It always helped to remember Luis's words—that despite physical evidence to the contrary, we are just fine. Much of that time, I was grateful that I could remember life's wisdom without actually dialing Luis's phone number. On occasion, I called him just to share how connected I felt to others and within myself.

Seamless Ties

beneath the body's surface
of immobility and pain
each molecule, cell, and neuron,
each weary breath,
hopeful tear,
and persistent will
orchestrate small steps
on shaky crutches
a radiant moon
animates the spirit
that propels love
that infuses mind

that feeds the muscles
that connects the body
to others —
charting the dance —
in gratitude

Yes, the gratitude was genuine, but as my body repaired, the financial arena unraveled. A debt of $50,000, which my health insurance did not cover, mounted daily. Insurance covered most doctor visits and treatments, but I paid the copayments. Medical complications plagued me for months after leaving the hospital. To address the problems with conventional medical interventions, I was limited to chemotherapy and steroids, which meant that I had to cover the full costs of all complementary medicine, including chiropractic, Chinese herbal treatment, and acupuncture, as well as therapeutic massage, all of which benefited me greatly. I did not feel grateful about the debt, yet a deeper part of me reminded me to remain trusting.

While looming financial pressures were stressful, I was making great progress in practicing a "one day at a time" approach. With every harassing phone call from the HMO billing office, I slipped into confusion and disarray. I thought I had to solve this problem alone, forgetting the earlier lessons that "I am not alone." During these worrisome moments, I couldn't help wondering, Why is it that in this culture we face so much aggravation just when we most need the assistance of an automatic safety net? All of these stressors occur during a time in people's lives when the support should be increased. Instead, insurance companies force us into becoming paper mongers, documenting, explaining, defending, and justifying every action. Friends reminded me to be grateful, given the millions of people who don't even have medical insurance.

Dealing with financial insecurity along with medical uncertainty drew me inward to the faith that had seen me through much fear, pain, and loss. This was no magic act. Choosing to see my situation from a perspective of wholeness meant doing some systematic reading from *A Course in Miracles Workbook* and doing the daily activities. In addition to spiritual practices, I also took proactive steps to educate myself on life's practical matters. I studied finance and developed a new attitude about money. Thoughts of insufficiency gave way to gratitude for every breath, every cent, and every loving person in my life — regardless of how things appeared to the contrary. I surrounded myself with resource books, workshops, and financial experts. Thankfully, family generosity, accompanied by lots of beans and tortillas, got me through the lean times of this transition period while I systematically downsized my expenses.

Without a doubt, money issues always stressed me more than anything else. That's not to say that all was smooth in other areas. An unexpected stress in what was already a tough time occurred when my trusted rheumatologist, Dr. Barrett, left her practice. Unwilling to continue in the intolerable HMO system, she closed her office. For seven years, she had been the expert in my case. I ached with fear, abandonment, and worry at the thought of having to start anew with a different specialist.

Getting out to interview doctors with whom I could work took every ounce of strength I could muster. Still unable to drive, I relied on Paratransit to shuttle me around the Bay Area in search of a doctor with whom I could collaborate. No longer did I expect doctors to cure me. However, I wanted a specialist to assist me in managing my health program, preferably a person knowledgeable in integrated medicine, where conventional and complementary medicines meet.

Searching for a new specialist was humiliating and exhausting. Carrying my heavy file of seven years of information about my treatment with Dr. Barrett, I now found myself in alienating offices, subjected to questions that reduced me to a specimen. Unlike my research travels to friendly communities, visits led to predictable frustration. Many doctors find working with patients with chronic illness frustrating. Some consultations with well-known neurologists and rheumatologists showed me the most unethical and uncaring side of medicine. As long as I remained peaceful, I could trust the process regardless of how exhausting it was.

One of the worst on the list of unsuitable doctors was a rheumatologist. Paratransit took me on crutches to my appointment at his office. I waited an hour until the receptionist called my name. Finally, the doctor came in to talk to me. He took my file and flipped through it as though he was reviewing a book in the bookstore. Three minutes later he looked up at me and without examining me said, "You need to get off the steroids. They're not helping you. I'll let your internist know." So I went off the medications, only to return to my internist two weeks later. He diagnosed me with a very inflamed liver and a suspicious rash.

"I'm calling the rheumatologist," he said.

"Why?" I asked.

"Because he may be able to offer some direction."

"That doesn't make sense," I told him.

"He said that I should discontinue the steroids and I did."

After a few minutes, the internist returned. "He says I should get you on the maximum level of steroids."

No way, I said to myself. I'm out of here. I didn't return to see either of them again.

On the other end of the spectrum of doctors I consulted was a very caring one. He asked me to send him my complete file so he could review it before my appointment. The appointment day arrived. I dreaded it. The doctor ended our meeting with, "You seem to be doing all that can be done through alternative medicine. I'm sorry, but allopathic medicine doesn't have much to offer people with your condition." That's the honest truth, I thought.

My experience through the ins and outs of traditional and alternative medicine made me think about the ideal service provider. It would be a "health manager," someone who could help me decide what type of healer or medical care would benefit me most. Given all of my experience, maybe that wise health manager was within me, waiting for me to listen for the next step. First, I needed lots of rest before resuming my quest internally and externally.

At times, the ordeal of interviewing potential doctors caused me great anxiety. Daily, in quiet meditation, I kept practicing what made sense to me in the face of continuous frustration. To maintain some sense of harmony, I had to keep remembering that there was more to me than the anguish of finding a new doctor. I relied on my friend Dr. Ralph Ortiz for chiropractic treatments. He had treated me for many years — without expecting payment when I could not pay. I appreciated his generous contribution to everyone's healing, since he has always been equally caring to all in his community.

More than half a year passed before I found a knowledgeable and caring ear willing to work with me. I had read an article about doctors of physical medicine and rehabilitation who worked with patients with chronic physical disabilities. In June 1997 I found Dr. Berry, a physiatrist, in the *Yellow Pages*! Dr. Berry specialized in physical medicine, rehabilitation, and immunology, encouraging the body to heal itself. I was impressed with this innovative specialist, whose training theory in healing was that the immune system could rebuild through natural and holistic treatment, including dietary supplements along with specialized physical therapies. After completing countless tests, she comprehensively analyzed my case. Nothing escaped Dr. Berry's attention. She addressed major problem areas, especially the depleted adrenals. Her action plan was to detoxify and strengthen the immune, muscle, and skeletal systems.

Immediately I trusted her, and we agreed to work together. She was the first doctor I had met since Dr. Barrett who listened to me and treated me as an intelligent adult who knew her own body and health history. She believed that she could help me even though, as she said, "You'll have to give me lots of time. After all, your problem has had years to get the way it is. It won't improve overnight." I burst into tears, already hopeful that it was possible for me to feel stronger.

Dr. Berry prescribed a daily, rigorous, muscle-strengthening physical therapy at home and a special physical therapy for soft tissue twice weekly at her office. The grueling, rolling motion on the deep tissue all over my back was intended to strengthen me but was tantamount to torture. Frequent nonsteroidal shots in the lower back, hips, and chest to ease the pain left me breathless. But all of it was worth it. Within a short time, I noticed easier mobility. Additionally, Dr. Berry prescribed a nutritional program, which included potent supplements and herbal regimens. Between breakfast and bedtime,

I took so many supplements that I dedicated an entire cupboard to them. None of this felt like an inconvenience; although Dr. Berry was a physician in the Western tradition, she spoke my language of healing. She encouraged and supported me to take full responsibility for my healing, including using multiple methods.

Along with Dr. Berry's biweekly physical therapies, I followed an intense Chinese medicine program of acupuncture, daily tai chi, and boiled herbs between meals. Rest, of course, was mandatory. The Chinese tradition has a good attitude about food. Chinese Medicine believes that foods are healing if we eat what our bodies want. Listening carefully to my body's wants dictated my diet. A refrigerator magnet held the list of stimulating, neutral, and calming foods, giving me plenty of choices, depending on how my body felt and what it craved. On warm summer days, my body craved cool, crisp carrots and ginger on a bed of lettuce. At the other extreme, when light fog and rain combined, I found myself in front of the stove, stirring up a pot of hearty chicken and vegetable soup with diced jalapeño peppers.

The healing process continued one breath at a time. I added Claramae Weber, a nurse and energy touch healer, to my team of healers. She helped me stay on a more even keel through her amazing hands-on energy work. Now my self-esteem and identity were less dependent on physical strength. I was less inclined to be hard on myself when I didn't accomplish personal or work goals. It became easier to embrace the light and dark within, making room for it all.

I also added Karyn Sanders, a stupendous herbalist whom I first heard on her KPFA radio program. Her holistic Native American herbal approach to healing and balancing one's inner strength with our external conditions made her a perfect fit philosophically. All of these efforts contributed to the continuously growing strength I was feeling day by day.

However, one problem that plagued me since the most recent severe relapse was reading. It had become an ordeal. Making sense of anything I read was extremely difficult. Reading a page three times became the norm. I couldn't retain a single word I read without enormous effort, much less comprehend an entire story. Frightening as it was, I adapted. A friend invited me to a meeting of her book group. The women were from diverse professional and ethnic backgrounds. It was refreshing to read books that I never had the time for when I was a professor.

The book group was special. I had never participated in a group where people were so respectful of each other's differing views. Sharing in engaging monthly conversations about books around a scrumptious home-cooked potluck made our meetings too enjoyable to miss even when I felt ill or embarrassed that I couldn't get through even one chapter. The group became a pivotal part of my healing community. I surrounded myself with nurturing people. They didn't judge me for what I believed or expressed.

We shared more than book discussions. Over the years, we've attended each others' parties, holiday dinners, a retirement dinner, wedding celebrations, and even the very unexpected memorial of a dear friend and a founding member of the group. The relationship bonds around books and life celebrations deepened as my body strengthened. Stretch by stretch, I felt stronger and stronger. Six months after I began working with Dr. Berry, I no longer needed the wheelchair. I had graduated to forearm crutches, and occasionally, just one cane.

Dr. Joyce, a family practice physician, became a key part of my healing team. Dr. Berry referred me to her because a family practice doctor had to make official referrals to specialists in order for me to get insurance coverage. Dr. Joyce supported complementary medicine. She listened compassionately and affirmed the healing program I had in place. She also recommended natural remedies for me to try before prescribing allopathic medicine. Whenever I visited, she always inquired about the physical therapists, acupuncturists, or other healers I worked with. As she always reminded me with a smile, "I can learn from you, too."

From west to east, medical modalities abound. I'm grateful to live in a part of the country where so many alternatives are available. Using a variety of healing modes strengthened my body. But the purpose was bigger. Each method helped me integrate the mind, body, and spirit.

Months following the acute relapse, I was strong enough to get behind the wheel of a car, hold on to the steering wheel, and step on the pedals long enough to drive myself around the block. Then I returned home, got my oxygen, and rested for the remainder of the day. The important thing was that it was one trip around the block more than yesterday. With confidence, I looked forward to driving around two blocks the next day. The *curandera*'s words rang from deep inside me: "Move forward from a place of faith and love."

CHAPTER 9

Finding Harmony

...love comes only as we find love within.
—bell hooks

As a child, I watched my mother strike a match and light a candle sitting in front of a saint she prayed to. It was a moment so sacred that I stopped what I was doing. The healing power of a candle has followed me. Every time I hold the taper to light a candle, I feel a balm filling me. Its grace empowers me. This very power is what a handful of healers have animated in me. Some don't have official titles, but I consider them healers because a word, a book, or a lifetime of love on their part influenced me to shift my perception of myself or of life. Consequently, the shifts I made because of these healers empowered me. Some of these relationships were lifelong; others were brief encounters. I admit that I didn't always appreciate the importance of their wisdom at the time, but when I reflected on them, there was no doubt as to the power of their influence.

One of the most challenging lessons came from the spiritual texts that Luis assigned for homework after each meeting. I read from numerous spiritual writings and wrote in my journal daily. The latter was already a familiar practice, but reading *A Course in Miracles* was more difficult because it was very abstract material. So I treated it like a new college course, taking notes as I went along and discussing them with Luis. Learning to do things differently stretched me out of a comfort zone, but I wouldn't have it any other way. Growing through study had been a lifelong thirst.

If accepting one's feelings without judgment was a way of becoming whole, I needed more evidence. It seemed easier to think that there were bad and good feelings and all I had to do was deny the bad ones. Now I was experiencing them all fully as Luis encouraged me to do. They felt miserably heavy, weighing on me like lead.

Countless calls to Luis reassured me that the intense feelings I had were quite healthy, even if some of them were anything but comfortable. The important part was that I experience them. Okay, so I knew that, but I needed someone to remind me often. Luis's explanations comforted me because I wanted so much to believe that the distressing feelings erupting within would pass. He made himself available to me twenty-four hours a day to talk. Sometimes I needed to, even though it went against my preference for working things out alone. Calling anyone, including Luis, broke my rules about self-sufficiency, but our phone sessions and occasional meetings got me through many crises.

Following each session, Luis's message stayed with me throughout the week. Still, most of my waking hours were devoted to working the body, and sometimes this burned me out. So on weekends, my attention turned to recreation and pleasing sounds for healing. I spent afternoons and evenings sitting at my favorite jazz clubs in San Francisco. Music spoke to me louder than any medical words.

Unfortunately, it didn't take much for university politics to stress me out of a harmonious frame of mind. One particular situation brought home just how insensitive institutions could be. Some colleagues from a university-appointed committee circulated a written internal review of our department, stating that because of my medical leaves, two professors in the division were having to teach more than their official load. I retorted with a well-crafted letter, explaining the committee's error in not considering my side of the story. First, I never took a medical leave. I had earned a sabbatical, and used only one quarter of it. The committee had failed to consult me about my colleagues' concerns, and had ignored my many efforts to continue teaching, researching, and performing university service. At the time of the report, I had only taken one quarter of medical leave in five years. The rest of the time, my breaks had been sabbaticals to conduct research and write academic manuscripts. Furthermore, throughout the illness, I had taught full-time despite all the obstacles the university put in my way. The truth was that no one had ever taught my classes during any of my sabbatical leaves.

I sent thirty letters to various colleagues across campus who had a part in the design and distribution of that committee report. Not one ever responded to my concerns and questions. Their silence was another form of their insensitivity. Nonetheless, I felt good about having asserted my position. It helped put things in perspective. I was taking charge clarifying, validating myself at a time when others opposed me. This was indeed a step forward.

At the end of my winter-quarter leave, this ordeal was

rewarded with a surprising accolade. The Spencer Foundation selected me to receive one of the highest awards given to senior scholars in my field. With the money the foundation gave me, I was able to continue meeting doctoral students. I funded five of my students to continue their research for two years. These five exceptional students and I became a close group of colleagues, shaping a dialogue on the meaning of scholarship in theory, practice, and in our personal lives. Our seminar meetings were rich with talk about our writings and humorous life stories that enlivened our ideas.

Family commitments tugged at me just as I wanted to focus on work. Mom's health waned. "Mom had a stroke," came my sister Lucy's voice over the phone. Immediately my own body's needs went on hold. In a matter of hours, I was on a flight to Los Angeles.

Over the years, Mom had met with obstacles from the medical system similar to those that people with chronic illnesses experience. Her health problems were dismissed when she didn't match the textbook case. In the Western tradition, physicians are trained to label the patient's problem according to the book and then find a cure for it. If the problem doesn't fit the textbook, the frustrated doctors consider it too much of a problem to partner with the patient to find workable holistic solutions. Over the years, I had seen Mom's doctors play the blame game when they couldn't identify the problem. "She's old," some said. Others described her problem as "chronic without a cure." I always wondered if they considered aging a chronic condition. Actually, blaming is the real illness. It's medical arrogance to think that people can control everything in their lives, including being healthy and becoming ill. Underneath such blaming is the fear of becoming ill ourselves. Medical providers are no exception; pointing the finger at those who don't respond to textbook treatments falsely insulates them from a similar fate.

After spending an exhausting week with Mom at the stroke center in the hospital, I returned home a few pounds lighter. Anxiety loomed as I wondered how long her strength would hold.

For Mom as well as for myself, I wanted to maintain the right perspective about healing. Most of my life, I had seen Mom work nonstop even when she was ill. One could say she was a poor role model for demonstrating ways to take care of one-self. However, her words to me about taking care of myself held important wisdom. In fact, she was saying, "Do as I say, not as I do." That was the message, which I took to heart when I set healthier limits. I was getting comfortable with the idea of creating flexibility in my schedule. That's the flexibility I appreciated in "Mexican time."

Whether in Mexican or any other time, there are spaces in our lives when we wish we could stop the clock to shield us from the pain of grief. Mom's suffering concerned me more than my own body's pain. Her health had deteriorated to the point of requiring full-time home nursing care. I had to be willing to let her go even though it would hurt. One sunny day, I called Mom at the nursing home where she had returned weeks earlier, thinking that a family member would answer. Not expecting to hear Mom, I was thrilled to talk to her, though her voice was faint and strained. She said that it had stopped raining in Whittier. The early weeks of that year had been soaked with relentless rain.

"The Bay Area is still drenched, Mom, but they predict dry weather by the middle of the week."

"It's beautiful here, *mi hija* (dear daughter). The flowers outside are so beautiful."

"I'm glad, Mom."

She sighed happily. "The flowers are so pretty, so pretty."

"Yes, Mom, I'm looking forward to seeing the sun here, too."

"Oh, you should see it, the colors are so beautiful, *mi hija*."

"I'm sure they are, Mom. I'll let you rest, and I'll call you tomorrow. I love you." After talking with her, I realized that Mom didn't have a view of any flowers from her room. Her window looked out on a parking lot. Mom's garden bloomed where only the soul could see.

One week later, on February 4, 1995, mild, gentle breezes finally reached the Bay Area. It made the day feel like springtime in winter. On the way home from a meeting with a colleague, I looked forward to calling Mom, whose last days were drawing near. As I walked into the house, I immediately checked the answering machine. It flashed eleven messages. Oh, God—I knew right away that Mom had died. It was true, and it felt so permanent. Part of me had believed that she would remain ill forever. Before her death, Mom and I had resolved the little wrinkles in our mother-and-daughter relationship. Now all I could do was pray for her to find peace and an end to her long, difficult journey. I pictured her walking among the beautiful flowers she had described in our last conversation.

In a space of timelessness, I sat up that night, unable to sleep. I wrote Mom a letter telling her how much I loved her, how I admired her courage and strength through her lifetime of struggle, her perseverance and total unselfish giving of herself to me, our family, and everyone she met. Even though I couldn't talk face to face with Mom again, the spirit of the letter would reach her. She would know how much I love her.

I called Berta. She asked what I needed. "Just someone to accompany me to buy a dress."

"Buy a dress?"

"Yes, Mom would want me to wear a new dress to her services."

Mom cared a great deal about her appearance and always dressed very nicely. Even when we were too poor to buy expensive clothes, she said, "*Uno tiene que presentarse bien. Aunque sean viejas las garitas, tienen que estar limpias.*" (One has to appear presentable. Even if your clothes are tattered, they need to be clean.) This was her time to be recognized and honored. She deserved a new dress!

Never before had I appreciated the miracle of life and death. This was different from the times when uncles, aunts, and cousins had died, when my parents made my sisters and me walk up to the coffin to pay our respects. As a child, I would approach the casket, trembling with fear that the dead would rise up and grab me. But Mom looked so peaceful in her coffin. She didn't look like Mom. Maybe it was because she really was no longer there. Now she just lived in me. Mom had suffered so much that I, too, felt peaceful for her.

My grief and emptiness weighed a ton. Mom was dead, but the thought that she was finally free sedated me momentarily. The question that haunted me was whether we had to die in order to be peaceful. I had to know.

"Not so!" Luis had reassured me, when I asked him about death. He underscored that the way to heal in this lifetime was to find a way to live peacefully on earth. "To think that peace lies anywhere else is to relinquish our power," he said. Some of these thoughts found their way into the eulogy I delivered on behalf of our family.

To tell about Mom's life was a joy in itself. Her innate modesty had shielded her tireless faith, which triumphed over hideous poverty as she raised five daughters to be professional women in a culture so different from hers. The intensity of her words to me when I was young, "Your best is good enough," sustained me on crutches in St. Mary's Church in front of the hundreds of people who attended the funeral mass. That was what she conveyed to me in her sometimes subtle and other times jarring ways—like dying. In twenty-five years of public speaking, I had never been so prepared and unprepared all at once. I realized that I was good enough. Mom knew that and now I accepted it.

On the day following her funeral, I went to Dad's house to be with him for a while. He had just returned from the cemetery and he was very upset. Evidently, the cemetery staff had cleared all of the flowers from Mom's gravesite. There must have been thousands of dollars' worth of flowers sent by all her family and friends. Dad stood in the dining room holding a ribbon. "Look, this is all I found there." The ribbon read, TO MY BELOVED WIFE. It had blown away from the spray of white carnations that covered mom's casket. Dad lowered his head and began sobbing quietly.

I hugged him, "Oh, Dad, I'm so sorry."

Buttoning up his emotions, he raised his head and proceeded to reveal the truth of his life. "I thought of going to complain and fight with the management at the cemetery, but I didn't have the energy. I spent all of my life trying to protect your mom and you girls, and I can't anymore. I'm tired." In tears, I watched my entire childhood flash before me. All of my childhood healed in one instant. All those years I thought Dad was just a gruff and strict father, but he was just playing his role as a father the best he knew—trying to protect us. Compassion filled my heart for this wounded old man who had done the best he could in the way he perceived his role as a father. This revelation deepened and strengthened our relationship profoundly until the end, five years later, when he was reunited with Mom.

When I think back on this moment of forgiveness between my father and me, I'm reminded of the continuous opportunities to heal. Every day in the face of sadness, grief, and confusion we can connect through love and forgiveness. These are the transformative moments when we can appreciate the perfection and purpose of our lives.

In the weeks following Mom's death, I still felt heavy with grief. I craved being alone. To avoid superficial conversations, I didn't answer the phone. In solitude, I surrendered to the hollow feelings, where only my higher power accompanied me, braiding the light and dark within. Discussing the enigmas of death with loved ones helped me to put it in some perspective. I was reminded of how something as natural as dying is sanitized in this society. Death is silenced as if we could escape it. We act as though it is the biggest secret, when in reality it is the one certainty we all share.

Mexican culture, like other cultures rooted in the truths of the earth, has a healthier outlook on death than more industrialized cultures, who often hide its reality from everyday life. Death is recognized and celebrated in Mexican art, music, and literature, it is even celebrated as a national holiday, *Día de los Muertos* (Day of the Dead). Every November 2, people in many towns in Mexico and in the US erect altars to honor the spirits of loved ones who have died. In celebration, we recognize our connection in spirit with those who have gone before us.

Traditionally, in Mexico, people wear black for a designated period of time, depending on which member of the family has recently died. The bereft are accorded respect, time, and space to grieve without having to make excuses for their emotions. In contrast, contemporary culture in the US values speed in mourning. Whenever there was a death in her family, Mom dressed in black for a year. She did that for her parents and brother. But as much as I like wearing black, I did not follow the custom for her. Instead, little by little, I reached out to loved ones to help me reconnect with life.

How we think about death, the loss, our emotions, how we dispose of the body and what happens to it, and how we remember our departed — all these are embedded in our cultural tapestry. In US society we tend to deal with death as a subject to be avoided at all costs, but we can still move through loss, grief, and pain to appreciate the true spirit and a person's life. Like other crises in a family, death can move us toward each other in love and forgiveness. Dad and I were an example; Mom's death brought us together.

Dad began reaching out to my sisters and me to talk about how things were going for him and to check in with us about the happenings in our lives. As new as this was for me to hear from him without Mom on the other end encouraging him to say hello, it felt loving. I looked forward to our phone chats. It was like wearing a new pair of shoes; they feel tight at first and maybe there's a sore spot in the heel, but the more they're worn, the more comfortable they become; they may even become a favorite pair.

For about a year, I flew down to Los Angeles monthly to visit my family, but I spent most of the time with Dad. We loved eating pancakes at Jack's, his favorite neighborhood restaurant.

We filled the weekend with more than pancakes. Our conversations were rich with family history: his childhood in a Mexican Yaqui Indian family, his working as a sheepherder, and raising of nine brothers and sisters, since he was the oldest, at thirteen when their father died. So, this was the story behind the strict, hardworking man I had grown up with. Suddenly his stern ways and work values made sense to me. This was the strength that both Mom and Dad modeled for us. I couldn't get enough of Dad's stories. I had found a new friend and a new father. Our precious time together was an unexpected gift after Mom's death.

Besides bonding with Dad, Mom's death also opened me to listening better with my heart where self-care mattered. Lots of bed rest at home, together with a gentle pacing of activity, quiet meditation and good nutrition occupied long hours. Self-care was the equivalent of a full-time job. Nonetheless, committing to living differently kept me focused on simple goals: looking out at my garden, walking down off the deck into the garden, and digging the soil to plant new seeds was enough.

When I first moved into my new home, the backyard had looked like an abandoned timberland. Part of the solution was easy; professional gardeners came to clear away the dead bushes. But like cultivating a healthy body, growing a robust garden was up to me. Every time Dad called, he asked for a progress report on the trees. "Dad, I have a lemon tree so prolific that I don't know when it's time to prune it."

"Prune it in the early months of the year."

"Okay, Dad." He knew a great deal about pruning trees. By spring of the following year, a semblance of life appeared in the backyard. Friends helped plant new daisies, camellias, and jasmine bushes.

The scent of night-blooming jasmine took me back to Grandma's house in Los Angeles, where I spent many summers. I can still hear the crickets chirping outside and see Grandpa and Grandma sitting in the living room listening to the evening news on the radio. A delicate fragrance of jasmine entered through the bedroom window. But Grandma's pride was her sturdy green *nopales* garden. Some grew in thick brown terra cotta pots while others stood stately against the back fence. Green *nopales* produce medicinal and nutritional benefits. The prickly tough exterior of the cacti protected their edible sustenence. So when Carmen came to visit me in my new home, I was delighted that she brought one of Grandma's potted cacti. It was a Mexican green rose succulent. I pictured Grandma smiling on the garden that was slowly taking shape.

Like grandma's succulents in the garden, I held my head up and put on a strong face for the physical therapist and even for myself. After a full afternoon of arduous physical therapy, I sat in my wheelchair, staring out the bedroom window, afraid that I wouldn't be able to care for myself. On a cool autumn day, I wondered, who is this woman who is wearing my clothes? In full view were the thirsty hydrangea bushes that no one had remembered to water. Suddenly, a soft voice reminded me that I was not alone. "I am taking care of you," it whispered in a strong but reassuring voice. Joyful tears streamed down my cheeks. They were the tangible imprint left by this messenger who had awakened my spirit twice before in the hospital. The powerful message epitomized all of the lessons on this healing journey—I am not alone.

After six months of leave from the university, I had a major decision to make. When the letter from the vice-chancellor arrived in the mail, my heartbeat and breathing accelerated, because I knew I wasn't ready to return to a full-time job. Her message was clear: if I could not return full-time as a professor, I had to surrender the position. By now, my health had improved some, but dealing with the demands of the work was still impossible.

Karen, a friend and colleague, listened to my story with a compassionate ear. She, too, had faced horrendous repercussions from the university when she became ill. After some thinking, I decided to propose to the university a new position in which I could minimize exertion and travel: I could teach from the UC Berkeley campus through interactive television, affording me more time to strengthen. The university rejected the proposal because it was too costly. There were no funds available for such a program.

I didn't have the stamina or presence of mind to fight the case. I resigned my position at the university. A couple of students offered to pack up my books and move me out. Devastated, I grieved over the loss of my identity as a professor and the security of a paycheck. For now, the uncertainty of my health made it impossible to pursue another career. There they were—my raw feelings exposed. Emptiness defined the long days that followed. But now I saw emptiness differently than in the past. It was a gift. The emptiness was an opportunity to learn something new and to open myself to new surprises.

Keep Dancing

In search of encouragement and inspiration, I attended a lecture by Oliver Sacks. A longtime fan of his writings, I could not pass up the opportunity. He was the keynote speaker at the UC Berkeley Forrester Lecture Series, where he discussed the patients in his book *Awakenings*. Following his talk, Sacks answered questions from the audience. I wrote my question: "How is it possible for the body to dance when unable to perform daily operations such as walking without supports?" On crutches, I joined a line, question in hand, waiting to hand it to the master of ceremonies. But by the time I arrived, I was last in line. I walked up to the stage and the emcee waved his hands—no more questions. I showed him my piece of paper as a thousand people listened to Oliver Sacks' parting words. Disappointed but resigned, I leaned against the wall, waiting until the applause ceased before I would walk to the back exit. As Sacks stepped back from the podium, the emcee took his arm, escorted him to the edge of the stage, and motioned me forward. Me? I pointed to myself. He nodded yes and waved again. Oliver Sacks shook my hand. I expressed a deep admiration of his work, then asked him my question. He asked about my problem, and then responded.

"Well, different parts of our brain operate different motor activities, and we don't know much yet about what I call performance. The power of performance and the concentration to hold someone together takes over. For many people, this performance ability is in control when they hear music. I'm beginning to write about this now. Those articles will be published soon."

"I'll look forward to reading your work on the topic."

"I wish you well. Whatever helps you move, do it."

I smiled and walked back up the aisle. Sacks' words animated me. His message to keep moving in whatever way my body felt good affirmed that healing spirit within me. His language encouraged me to do what I loved. I could keep moving through dance, despite all the pain.

Sacks believed that the important question is not what disease you have. Rather, it is what person has the disease. By reversing the question, we place the emphasis on our self-ability. I wanted to tap that place of peace as I healed not only physically but emotionally.

As profound as the grief felt after departing from the university, a call from Carmen sank me into an even deeper sorrow: "Thought you should know that the paramedics just took Dad to the hospital because he had a major heart attack." Suddenly I felt trapped in a thick, dark cloud of anxiety.

"Oh, my God. Should we fly down now or wait?" I asked.

Carmen quickly added, "It doesn't look good. I'll make reservations for a flight down for both of us."

"Okay. Just let me know what time you'll pick me up."

True, Dad was not young, but he seemed in pretty good shape. He had walked about five miles daily since moving into the retirement apartment. I felt heavier with every worrisome thought of what would happen.

Hours later that evening, we five sisters gathered outside of Dad's room in the intensive care unit. Without a family member present to intervene, Dad had been resuscitated when he arrived in the hospital, and had been placed on a respirator and other life-support units. His situation seemed hopeless, and the doctors wanted our decision about removing him from life support. The emotional burden was now up to us, his daughters, to execute his health directive and remove him from artificial means of sustaining life. Dad's doctor coached us on the most medically appropriate time that Dad could be removed from life support, and every morning he gave us a report on Dad's situation. My sisters and I held vigil in the waiting room and on the floor outside his room. On crutches, I walked up and down the hallways. We cried, told stories about Dad, ate chocolate truffles, and waited for the inevitable. At night, we took turns going home to rest for short periods.

After five days, the time arrived to let Dad go. The doctor reported that Dad was now at the point of no return. He recommended that we gather the family and let Dad continue making his transition. All of us had made our peace in the respective religious traditions we practiced. As the doctor removed the tubes and needles, we wept softly. We stood around the bed, watching Dad lie peacefully under the snowy white sheet.

Suddenly, without warning, Dad sat up, looked around at us, and in a deep, raspy voice, asked, "What happened?"

The doctor turned whiter than Dad's sheet. He looked at me and said, "This is nothing short of a miracle."

We stood in shock, then moved close to Dad's face, reassuring him. "Dad, we love you. We're here. Everything is fine. You just rest."

The doctor called Carmen outside the room and told her that sometimes after patients are removed from life support, they wake up for a brief time and then slip away quietly. He suggested that we all leave so that they could sedate Dad, since he seemed confused and agitated. They would have to observe him during the night to see what was happening. Of course, if he had cardiac failure or other organ failure, the next time they could not intervene at all.

What a mysterious thing death is, I thought as I lay awake staring at the ceiling that night. Would Dad die that night as the doctor predicted? Would he live on? How much longer? Maybe he had more things he wanted to do in this life. How would we ever know when we are through living our life's mission?

Anxious to know what was happening, at 6:00 a.m., Carmen

and I drove to the hospital, which was three miles away. We walked up to Dad's room in the intensive care unit, but the room was empty. We feared the worst: Dad had died and the doctor hadn't notified us. We couldn't find a familiar face on the floor to explain what had happened to Dad until several minutes later, when the regular nurse assumed her shift. She checked the records and told us, "Your father was moved to the cardiac ward on the second floor directly below this unit." She then apologized that no one had notified us.

Relieved, we couldn't get there fast enough. Even on crutches, I felt like I was flying. We couldn't imagine what state we would find Dad in. The big question we asked ourselves: Is Dad improved or stable? Finally, we arrived at room 202. We entered and found Dad in the bed closest to the door. He was sitting up, dressed in a short-sleeved, blue gown loosely tied around his neck. He sipped the cup of liquid he held, and he laughed as he watched an old *I Love Lucy* rerun. He saw us enter and pointed to the TV, laughing and mumbling something in garbled speech. We hugged him, and the nurse entered to tell us that they needed to administer a breathing treatment.

We stepped outside and caught the attention of his attending doctor. "How is Dad? What can we expect now?" Carmen asked.

The doctor responded, "He's doing amazingly well. But we don't know if he'll remain stable. We'll keep him here a few days and administer therapies to help him strengthen. Let's see how he does."

Three days later Dad was moved to the same convalescent facility where Mom spent time after her stroke. Dad befriended one of his roommates, Sammy, a Mexican man who spoke Spanish. He was a retired minister and the first friend I ever knew

Dad to have. He loved chatting and spending time with Sammy. I visited him on weekends and called him every evening. Our conversations were always in Spanish. The model patient, Dad followed his doctor's instructions. Dad spent hours in physical therapy each day. This eighty-five-year-old man stretched and choreographed his way to complete recovery in three weeks. On the night before he was to be released, I called him.

"Dad, you've really performed miracles in these three weeks. I'm drawing inspiration from you every day."

"I still don't know what happened, but I had lots of people helping me to get better."

"I hear you're going back to your apartment."

"Yes, *mi hija*, I'm ready to go home," he said.

Dad sounded peaceful. Then he talked about one of my aunts. He had just learned that she had died two weeks before. "I'm glad that she died peacefully," Dad said. "That's the best we can do."

"Yes, I guess we all want that."

"Don't forget to prune that lemon tree," Dad added. He always gave me some bit of advice on how to care for the car or the house.

"I'll do that, Dad. I love you."

"Me too, *mi hija*."

That was the last time Dad and I talked. Two hours later, my sister Marie called. "Dad had a massive heart attack and they took him to the hospital. He had enough time for the daughters and grandchildren to gather around his bed. He told us all he loved us and that he had to go."

"He had to do it his way," I said. "He wouldn't have it any other way."

Marie added, "You might want to know that when Dad had

the heart attack, he was in bed in his room. When the paramedics carried him out, he told Sammy to pray for him. Together they prayed as he was taken to the hospital."

"Dad finally made a good friend," I said. "It's the best kind of friend, who prays with you when you're dying."

During Dad's last weeks of life, the most important lesson he taught us was that we're never too old to transform our lives and to live to the fullest, even if it's just for a life-altering few weeks.

In the months that followed Dad's passing, I missed him so much. The same man who was the stern authoritarian during our early years had become my best friend after Mom died. Gratitude abounded as I recalled our weekend breakfasts and conversations about our family history. He left my sisters and me a great legacy of hard work, determination, love for family, discipline, good family stories, and at the end, the value of friendship.

I found myself in a place between no longer and not yet. Mostly, I stayed home, treasuring some time alone to grieve for Dad. In the hurricane of feelings, I also wanted quiet spaces to appreciate the freedom from the stress of my former job, even though I still felt the loss of leaving the university. When I felt more sociable, I accepted visits from family and friends.

Faith led me forward along with the loving spirit of those who had helped me to heal. I meditated on what kind of job I would get when I was able to work. In that quiet space, I made peace with knowing that I was not more than my feelings. Trusting that somehow I would be taken care of diminished the stress of wondering what my next job would be. Letting go of feeling as if I were a victim freed me to look forward to new opportunities. One warm, sunny morning I awoke and looked out to the deck, where Grandma's potted succulents sat. I felt especially tranquil, free from the worry and fear of "not having a direction." I knew exactly what I wanted: to heal my body and have a career that would allow me to remain strong. I felt entirely confident that I could do it. I felt fully deserving of having it.

Work meant different things now. I would no longer push my body until it collapsed. How I worked was as important as what I did. I was in a position to recommit to a new career, with my health as a top priority. One of Mom's favorite sayings, *Cuando Dios cierra una puerta, abre otras* (When God closes one door, He opens others), had never been so true.

Without a master plan, I took one day at a time. Every morning, after completing a physical therapy workout, I reclined in bed with the PowerBook computer on my lap. The Internet became my office. I went to online writing classes and reinvented my professional skills to include technical, professional, and nonfiction writing. Through e-mail, I stayed connected with friends and colleagues across the country. I began getting contracts to write for private and nonprofit industries. I stepped into new worlds, including environmental policies and community public health. I found myself immersed in exciting new subject areas and professional networks. When I had a spare minute, I turned to writing books about the communities in which I had worked as a researcher and advocate. My healthy bank account was the tangible measure that I was on the right track. For all of this I was grateful.

Nothing helped as much as long periods of rest. Unable to sit up for long, I alternated physical therapy with rest and more stretching. The routine strengthened me. With each strong step I took, my new career unfolded. From a newly organized home office, I learned new technical programs like Java and

Unix, which years before I would have guessed were either gourmet coffees or endangered species.

On the more creative end, I turned a new page into the world of writing classes, writing coaches, video documentary workshops, of nonfiction writer's weeks, book agents, and book doctors. Imagine my surprise in learning that even books have doctors. This new business also meant a renewed commitment to forging a personal literacy that could read the body's rhythm and shape a career to match. Though this didn't mean the end of research or of working in and with communities, it moved me away from the university and into the world of independent writing.

While transitioning to a new career, I kept some connections to academic projects, which I loved. One of those projects was writing the story of communities in which I worked. In the year 2000, my new book, *The Power of Community*, was published. It chronicled fifteen years of collaborative work and transformation in the lives of Carpinteria families. Although writing the book was an arduous undertaking while keeping up physical treatments and working on other technical writing, the families' lives inspired me to transcend all obstacles.

That same year, the Council on Anthropology and Education of the American Anthropological Association honored me with the George and Louise Spindler Award. George and Louise Spindler founded the field of anthropology and education in the 1950s. The field focuses on issues of learning in families, communities, and schools from a cultural perspective. George and Louise were also my professors at Stanford, which made the award even more special. The engraved plaque read: "In recognition of your distinguished and inspirational lifetime contributions to Anthropology and Education."

The audience in the packed grand ballroom at the San Francisco Hilton Hotel gave me a standing ovation when I walked up to receive the award on that chilly December evening. It was an unexpected, yet wonderful accolade for doing work that I love.

I focused on technical and creative nonfiction stories. This stretched unknown parts of me into the new millennium. Of the different writing that I have done, writing life stories of people with whom I have worked who transformed their lives and communities for social justice inspired and deepened me most. When my stories were accepted to the Hurston / Wright Writer's Week, it was particularly special because I had long admired Zora Neale Hurston's anthropological and literary works. I had the opportunity to work with excellent writers like Junot Diaz, Quincy Troupe, and Chitra Divakaruni, who taught workshops during that week. I began working with some talented Bay Area writers on a regular basis. Sande, a gifted artist and writer, was one of the best gifts of the Hurston/Wright Writer's Week. We became fast friends and supported each other's writing endeavors.

A new career and stronger health also encouraged me in the relationship arena, and I began dating again. In the past, expressing deep feelings in relationships with men had been difficult. Blaming my partner was the convenient thing to do. The challenge was to commit to myself in the relationship as much as to the other person—not in a selfish "you or me" opposition, but taking responsibility for my happiness in the relationship. In her book *Communion*, bell hooks has it right: "... love comes only as we find love within. To risk self-knowledge is to begin love's journey."[4] I guess it doesn't matter how long it takes us to awaken, that we wake up is what's important.

As important as dating was, so was playtime with friends. During tough times, they had helped me cook, shop, and clean house. They had provided transportation, and held my hand. Now that I was a bit more mobile, they wanted to me go out with them even though I was still getting around on crutches and canes. Whenever I had the energy, I couldn't resist their invitations to jazz clubs, movies, festivals, and parties. Shirley, a dear friend, knew that I loved dancing. She called one Monday, inviting me to meet her and other friends on Wednesday evening at a dance club. Wednesday was women's night and we'd get free admission. I could think of nothing better to celebrate just being able to get out.

Having rested for nearly two days in preparation for a night of dance, I grabbed my cane and went to meet a few friends at the hall. When the live salsa band began to play, a man approached our table.

He asked if I wanted to dance. "Yes, of course," I smiled.

"Didn't I see you walk in using a cane?" he asked on our way to the dance floor.

"I'm giving it a rest right now."

"Okay, well, let's salsa."

"Tonight I'm celebrating feeling good."

"You certainly look wonderful, and you're a great dancer."

I felt like a young girl at her first dance. I danced one entire dance, then I picked up my cane and kissed my friends goodnight. The warm salsa rhythms faded in the background as I walked slowly out the door. On the way home, memories of former tireless dancing marathons filled me. This was a one-dance night followed by three days of complete bed rest, shoulder-to-toes pain, and total debilitation. It was painful, but that one dance was good medicine for the soul.

The power of staying open to all possibilities changed my small world after the monumental catastrophe of September 11, 2001, the day the world changed. I talked with many friends all day long. In the evening, our church opened its doors for us to get together, share our impressions of the day, and pray.

Following the gathering, my friend Dudley and I talked for almost two hours about everything that was important to us. We had known each other for several years as members of the same church. I found him very easy to talk with. Afterward, I thought he might be interested in joining me at dinner at a Nepalese restaurant to celebrate my niece's twenty-first birthday. Confusion ensued between phone calls and e-mails so that by the time he called me, the dinner celebration had passed.

Although my initial reason for contacting Dudley had passed, he invited me to have dinner with him the following weekend. That was our first date. It was impossible to ignore the background of upheaval and tragedy on the world stage that shared a personal and historic time. For me, however, the transformative events in my world were exactly the opposite. Dudley awakened new feelings, changing what had been a casual friendship to a more serious relationship that blossomed day by day.

Dudley's story was set in the stability of his identity as an Iowan guy. In a short time, I learned what his strong connection to Iowa meant. His character told it all: he was a loving, intelligent, confident, hardworking, trustworthy person, and a lot of fun.

Not only were our romantic times totally special, but the difficult moments and events we shared also matured our relationship; this confirmed my strong feelings about him and about the relationship. More important, I grew into a deeper part of myself as commitment in a relationship became more possible. What made Dudley a completely different life partner was that he believed in my strengths and supported me through self-doubts and difficult times.

Dudley made it easy and a pleasure for me to reciprocate. He made it safe to be me whether I was with him or by myself. I had a new sense of me as a strong woman in a committed relationship. More than ever before, bell hooks' words felt true: the biggest risk in a relationship is our self-discovery.

We grew closer through tender moments as well as when some difficult obstacles confronted us. What confirmed this for both of us was that regardless of how difficult a situation was, we turned toward each other instead of running in the opposite direction. It was evidence that love was not two halves trying to become one. Rather it was two people, each entirely whole.

On a warm October evening, two years after our first date, Dudley and I married before 200 family members and friends. The effortless love, joy, and commitment that defined our relationship convinced me that this was the right step to take. At a reception in our backyard, we danced to the sounds of Rolando Morales-Matos' jazz combo. No canes or forearm crutches were necessary for our first dance.

CHAPTER 10

Honoring Lessons Learned

*I'm challenged by the notion that it's not what happens to us
that is important; it's how we deal with it that matters.*

I have come to understand that the primary source of
health is our inner power. Health, like illness, orchestrates
many parts of our life. Realizing that my body was destructible opened my heart to the indestructible. Healing demanded
that I transport myself back to my childhood to retrieve the
familial and cultural strengths I needed to empower myself.
I looked inward, crafting a healing language with faith, gratitude, forgiveness, love, and harmony at its center. In that way,
I came to believe that in the illness lies its own cure. Pain has
a voice. If we listen, we are given instructions on how to move
in the direction of healing.

Getting healthy became full-time work, not only because of
the chronic nature of the illness, but also because health is not
an end but a process, an adjustment of a whole life through spirituality, community, and recreation. It is not about relying on
external remedies. It is living from that place in me that keeps
me feeling grateful, faithful, joyful, stronger, and healthier.

On this voyage, the meaning of the word "healing" expanded to mean something much broader than merely fixing the physical symptoms. I learned that, contrary to our belief, the body does not have a mind of its own. A strong relationship exists between our body, mind, and spirit. It does seem easier for us to think about merely repairing the body or getting it to function in a healthy way. In reality, though, our perception of our physical environment, our perception of self, our understanding of the social systems we participate in, and how connected or disconnected we feel to our inner self all influence our overall health. We are more than our physical presence. We are integrated beings, spirit, body, and mind. As a whole person, I exercise more power when I heal not only the body but the soul.

I have been fortunate to have healers appear in many packages, working their cures in their own particular way. They may not have considered themselves healers, but to me they have all been pearls along the way. They include my parents, Dudley, my sisters, Luis and Patty, Berta and other special friends, Dr. Barrett, Dr. Berry, Dr. Ralph, Oliver Sacks, the acupuncturists, and the *curanderas* in communities where I have lived and worked. These people have challenged me to unfold my fullest potential as a person. They have taught me a key lesson—that we are never alone.

Many of the healers who have helped me physically are experts in Eastern and Western traditions. Others have played a more central role as totally supportive helping hands, my community of angels. Still others have been the flickering candlelight in dark times and catalysts in transforming feelings of helplessness to empowerment. Each in his or her unique way has kept me focused on healing by an encouraging word in a painful moment, by teaching me to see myself connected to Spirit, and through a lifetime of inspiring examples.

Although we could all agree that we want to have good health, I found myself asking a critical question: who is responsible for our wellness? Before I became ill, I had one answer: I believed that the doctor had full control of my well-being. Whenever I became ill, I couldn't get to the doctor fast enough to demand the strongest pills or medications available.

After navigating multiple healing modalities and traditions, I changed my answer to the question of who is responsible for our healing. Part of that responsibility meant that I had to ask my health providers the important questions in order to understand both of our roles in my care. Approaching an illness from a position of wholeness gave me control over my body. I became my strongest advocate as a researcher, manager, and caretaker. As the health crisis unfolded, I experienced fear, anger, and frustration. Then, I learned to quiet myself and listen to what the illness was telling me. My body became my teacher. Drawing from all the lessons along the way, I learned the following:

- I learned to trust my ability beyond its physical strength.

- Without a language to think and talk about our situation, we cannot give either illness or healing a voice. We need to speak about illness, about potential for healing, and about building supportive communities around us to transform our lives. By giving voice to our condition and listening to others, we gain awareness and access to choices and possibilities for healing.

- Stretching my physical, emotional, and spiritual muscle, I discovered the power of re-creation.

- When we can make decisions about our bodies and our lives, we are empowered. In that way, we transform our experience from that of victim to one of empowerment.

- Miracles are not things we wish for, they are inspired by our freedom from fear. It is not what happens to us that's important; it's how we deal with our problems that makes the difference.

- I'm challenged by the opportunity to see that there are no easy answers to important questions. To think that peace lies anywhere else but within us, is to relinquish our power.

- The best kind of friend is one who prays with you when you're dying.

- *Cuando Dios cierra una puerta, abre otras* (When God closes one door, He opens others).

- I have come to believe that in illness rests its own cure.

The prickly parts of my life are now easier to handle because I can cut through to the core. Rough spots overwhelm me less than before. The road I've traveled has taught me to respond more calmly when flare-ups occur. Although discouragement tugs at me when I feel unwell, it's easier to walk through the difficult times. With the aid of hindsight, I see that healing is a vehicle of possibilities for us to shift our perspective from separation to oneness.

Never would I have imagined that an illness that weakened

me so severely would be the catalyst for strengthening my inner voice. A healthier relationship with myself and loved ones is a testament to this. The writer Margiad Evans says, "Our health is a voyage and every illness is an adventure story."[5] Nothing catches our attention like pain and illness. So why not use them to move forward in our journey of self-discovery?

Realizing that a body is more than a machine and chemical apparatus, I began paying attention to the messages that came through the pain, fatigue, and other complications. Although many of us are born with vulnerabilities that undermine our health, I recognized that I had put my life out of balance. I was always too busy to listen to the warning signs. Buddha is said to have taught, "Our body is precious. It is a vehicle for awakening. Treat it with care." Since there is no separation between our body, mind, and spirit, we do need to take care of our bodies and to listen to the warning signs that can alert us. When we engage all of our being in our healing, we are acting from the part of ourselves that is whole—that part that speaks to us.

Illness has a built-in compass. Through it, we can discover who we really are. It can lead us to meeting people and traveling roads where we might not have gone had we not become ill. What better balm than to have ourselves as our own best friend in times of trouble, someone to tell us to rest, to slow down, to laugh, to forgive and to be grateful. Prior to the illness, impatience was more my style. But from the rubble, I began to piece together new visions that gave voice to another new language, this time a language of healing. Healing has given way to more enduring connections in my life. I've learned patience with myself where health and work are concerned.

I am also in a committed, loving marriage such as I've never known before. I can put work in perspective so that it doesn't defeat me; I don't have to wait until I'm in crisis to stop. I can listen to that wise healer in me daily. More important, I can draw on my faith every day, in gratitude. There is no greater gift than to trust a higher power through the light and darkness of life.

The ending here is another beginning for me. I am appreciative of every morning I can awaken to the light of day. Most days, before I get down to work, Dudley prepares our coffee. I get myself out of bed, walk around the neighborhood, wave to the neighbors, and occasionally chat with people like Sandy, whose garden contains the lush apple tree that is the midpoint of my daily walk.

As I turn the corner, walking back home, I'm lost in thought about the inspirations that shape my life: Faith, family, and friends form a loving community that keeps me balanced. They have helped me learn some of the lessons inherent in the illness, as well as the new language of gratitude, forgiveness, and joy. With gratitude, forgiveness follows. With forgiveness, joy emerges.

Fifteen years later, that joy brought Sandy and me together on a tranquil, sunny morning. Our bodies had parallel histories. We realized that our connection held years of pain and the struggle of dealing with autoimmune diseases. Now, that same body choreographs my daily walks around that house with the prolific apple tree.

Notes

1. In his book, *The Wounded Storyteller: Body, Illness, and Ethics*, Arthur W. Frank discusses the notion of quest narratives, which he says is about discovering how illness can be transformed into an experience whereby the person becomes someone new. (Chicago, IL: University of Chicago Press, 1995).

2. Stephen Levine. *Unattended Sorrow: Recovering from Loss and Reviving the Heart.* (New York: Rodale Books, 2005).

3. Mary Catherine Bateson. *Peripheral Visions: Learning Along the Way.* (New York: HarperCollins, 1994), p. 79.

4. bell hooks. *Communion: The Female Search for Love.* (New York: HarperCollins, 2002).

5. Margiad Evans in *Spiritual Literacy: Reading the Sacred in Everyday Life.* Frederic and Mary Ann Brussat. (New York: Scribner, 1998).

References

I have drawn inspiration from or referenced the following sources:

A Course in Miracles, Text. New York: Foundation for Inner Peace, 1975.

Anzaldua, Gloria. *Borderlands — La Frontera: The New Mestiza.* San Francisco: Spinsters/Aunt Lute, 1987.

Arrien, Angeles. *Signs of Life: The Five Universal Shapes and How to Use Them.* Sonoma: Arcus Publishing Co., 1992.

Bateson, Mary Catherine. *Peripheral Visions: Learning Along the Way.* New York: HarperCollins, 1994.

Brussat, Frederic and Mary Ann. *Spiritual Literacy: Reading the Sacred in Everyday Life.* New York: Scribner, 1996.

Cook, Marshall. *Slow Down and Get More Done.* Cincinnati: S&W Publications, 1996.

Delgado Gaitan, Concha. *Protean Literacy: Extending the Discourse on Empowerment.* London: Falmer Press, 1996.

Dossey, Larry. *Healing Words.* San Francisco: Harper San Francisco, 1993.

Duff, Kat. *The Alchemy of Illness.* New York: Bell Tower, 1993.

Frank, Arthur. *The Wounded Storyteller: Body, Illness, and Ethics*. Chicago: University of Chicago, 1995.

Frankl, Viktor. *Man's Search for Meaning*. New York: Pocket Books, 1963

Estés, Clarissa Pinkola. *Women Who Run With the Wolves*. New York: Ballantine Books, 1992.

Galeano, Eduardo (with Jose Francisco Borges). *Walking Words*. New York: W. W. Norton & Co., 1997.

Griffin, Susan. *What Her Body Thought*. San Francisco: Harper San Francisco, 2000.

hooks, bell. Communion: *The Female Search for Love*. New York: William Morrow, 2002.

Murphy, Robert F. *The Body Silent*. New York: W. W. Norton, 1987.

Neumann, Anna, and Penelope Peterson (Eds.). *Learning From Our Lives: Women, Research, and Autobiography in Education*. New York: Teachers College, Columbia University, 1997.

Radziuna, Eileen. *Lupus: My Search for a Diagnosis*. Alameda: Hunter House, 1989.

Rinpoche, Sogyal. *The Tibetan Book of Living and Dying*. San Francisco: Harper San Francisco, 1994.

Rumi (translated by John Moyne and Coleman Barks). *Say I Am You*. Athens: Maypop, 1994.

Sacks, Oliver. *An Anthropologist on Mars*. New York: Alfred A. Knopf, 1995.

Sanford, Agnes. *The Healing Gifts of the Spirit*. New York: HarperCollins Publishers, 1966.

Talman, Donna Hamil. *Heartsearch: Toward Healing Lupus.* Berkeley: North Atlantic Books, 1991.

The Boston Women's Health Collective. *Our Bodies Ourselves: Updated and Expanded.* Gloucester: Peter Smith Publisher, Inc., 2005.

Wallis, Velma. *Two Old Women: An Alaska Legend of Betrayal, Courage and Survival.* San Francisco: Harper San Francisco, 1993.

Wells, H. G. "*In the Country of the Blind.*" London: Nelson, 1910.

Williamson, Marianne. *A Return to Love.* San Francisco: HarperCollins Publishers, 1992.

Zohar, Danah. *The Quantum Self: Human Nature and Consciousness Defined by the New Physics.* New York: Quill/William Morrow, 1990.

About the Author

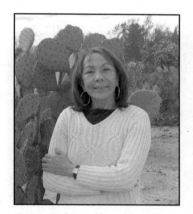

Concha Delgado Gaitan is an award-winning ethnographic researcher and writer of oral and written traditions in immigrant communities, including family and community empowerment through literacy. She has worked with Latino, Southeast Asian, Russian Refugee, and Alaskan Native communities in the US. Delgado Gaitan describes the empowerment of families, communities, and schools in her many publications, among them her seven books: *Culturally Responsive Classrooms; Involving Latino Families in the Schools; The Power of Community; Literacy for Empowerment; Protean Literacy; Crossing Cultural Borders; and School and Society.* Although it is in a different genre, her new book, *Prickly Cactus*, illustrates the role and strength of one's community, a concept that has defined her work from the beginning, as a professor of Anthropology and Education at the University of California, Santa Barbara and UC Davis.

Delgado Gaitan has also worked in the field of public health in culturally diverse communities. Her most recent academic interests involve applying public health and cultural theories to educational and social justice issues in society. Currently, Delgado Gaitan is a Visiting Professor at the University of Texas, El Paso. An avid walker, reader, and cook, she loves hanging out with family and friends when she is not lecturing or researching in other parts of the country. Delgado Gaitan is a writer in the San Francisco Bay Area where she lives with her husband, Dudley Thompson, and their tabby cat Sofia.